Golden Nuggets of Mercy

Patricia Brown
(Noble Brun)

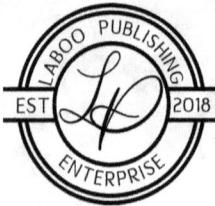

Table of Contents

Preface

"You can't get blood out of a turnip" is an idiom that describes a difficult task or situation that seems impossible to fix. In experiencing the severest of life's trials, one can be catapulted to a level of desperation in seeking a way out. Out of the varying responses and approaches to urgent crises, I chose to commit to a deeper relationship with the Almighty God of the universe. I have learned through my Christian experience that God through His word the Bible can guarantee that any problem encountered will work out for my good. Trusting Him and His Word was my first priority in approaching a terminal diagnosis.

Between these pages are words of inspiration and messages of love and encouragement focusing on everyday experiences. In reaching out to, and thinking of the needs of others, there was no time to worry about dying. Each month from the day of diagnosis (2011-2020) there is something penned that the reader can relate to and or learn via my experiences. I pray that your perusal, particularly among the Myeloma community, will brighten your outlook on what God can do through you in the midst of trials and trying times,

The Road Less Traveled

"The Road Not Taken" was one of my favorite works by American poet Robert Frost. Born in 1874, he was considered a modernist writer of his time, driven to extend his works beyond the traditions. I was in the tenth grade when I committed this poem to memory. It served as motivation to make right choices in life successful outcomes.

Around the age of 24, I gave my heart to the Lord, to serve him for the rest of my days. In my growth process I came across a passage similar to "The Road Not Taken." Matthew 7:13-14: "Enter in at the straight gate, for wide is the gate and broad is the way, which leads unto life, and few there be that find it."

The end of the poem reads, "Two roads diverged in a wood, and I took the one less traveled by, and that has made all the difference." It's always good to make right choices for success. However, the greatest choice is choosing Eternal Life, a road that is straight and narrow and less chosen by many. Make it right. Don't follow the masses. Repent and give Jesus your heart today. "For God so loved the world that he gave his only begotten son that whosoever believes in him should not perish but have everlasting life." #redeemingthetime

St. John 3:16

Watch Your Tongue

Thank you, Lord, for guidance. Thank you for the gift of the Holy Spirit. Thank you for putting a watchman at the door of my mouth that I might not sin against you. Forgive me for hurtful words. You have my heart. You have my tongue. Let my words bring healing. I don't want to say a word, unless it points the world back to you.

There are so many opinions expressed concerning what's happening in our nation and the world today. Opinions can be said in love, or can express hatred, cause separation and incite harm. "Let the words of my mouth and meditations of my heart always be acceptable in your sight." (Psalm 19:14, KJV) #rededemingthetime

The Harvest

Father, the harvest has been ripe, but the laborers have been few. Forgive us for our lack of diligence and concern for the lost. Restore our commitment, our joy and love to you and the commission whereunto you have called us. Many souls have fallen prey to the adversary and the plan to discredit your word, work and purpose in the earth. The world has consistently, through many generations and eons of time, gone backwards together. I woke up this morning grieved at the current conditions in the world, barely holding back tears over the same. I ask for your mercy today and going forward for the lost souls who have slipped through the gaps of prayer, those who have hardened their hearts toward the church, as well as those whose minds are blinded and refuse the truth of your word.

Father, intervene! My heart can barely take all the death and dying happening at every level, especially to the children, born and unborn. I have not read in your word some of the horrors that are happening in the earth today—the harvesting of organs for profit and murder for sport, just to name a few. You forgave your chosen people many times over by your mercy when they cried out to you for forgiveness. Forgive us this day, your body of Christ all over the world. Intervene in the madness that is overtaking the earth in this land and across the seas. The narrow road to your kingdom is becoming narrower and straighter. Let your hand of mercy be stretched out still to those who know not what they do. In the name of Jesus Christ our Savior, do

I submit my petition, urging all of my brothers and sisters to do the same. #redeemingthetime

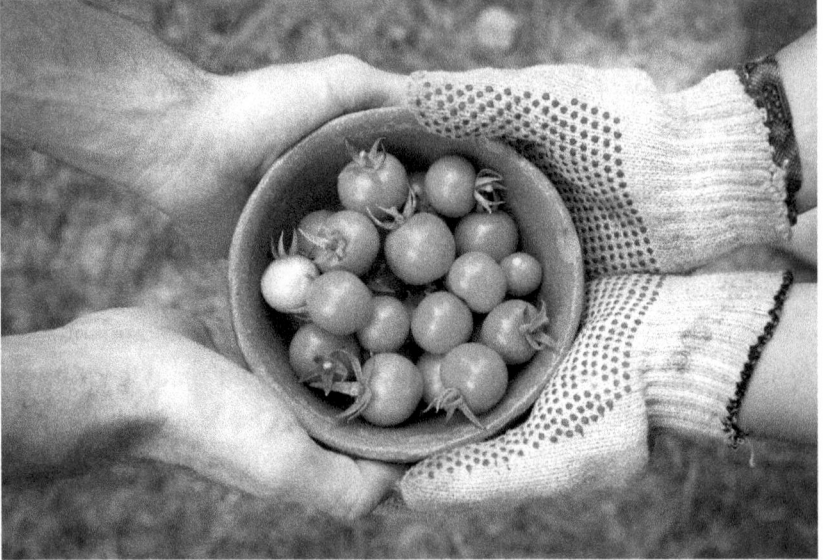

A Call For Prayer

Prayer changes things and people. In light of recent news events involving Syria and the killing of its own people, including children and babies, I am moved and shaken in my spirit to fervently pray and understand why. It's hard to look the other way when you actually see the suffering. Via breaking news, and a special report, a military strike by the U. S. was just ordered on that country. And upon checking reliable news sources, there are many issues involving several countries and their reluctance to get involved that play a part in this ongoing crisis. It helps to know what to pray for when asking God to make changes. Check your reliable news sources and join me in prayer. THIS IS NOT A POLITICAL POST FOR OPINION AND TALKING POINTS, BUT A CALL FOR PRAYER #comequicklylordjesus!

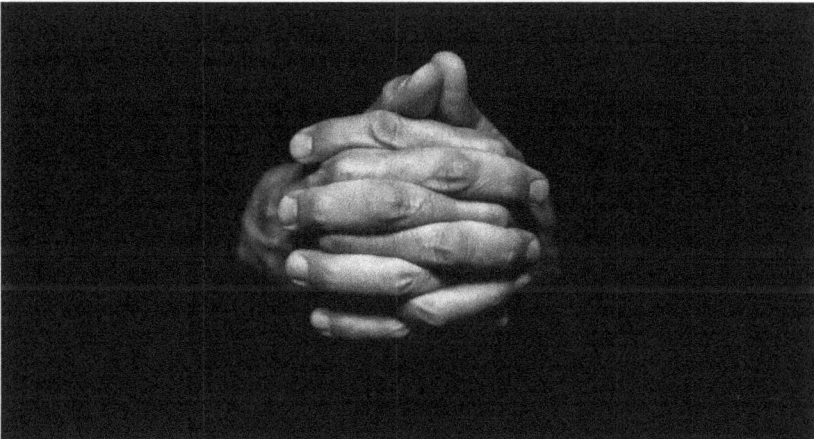

Animal In God's House

"Elephant in the room" is an English metaphor for an obvious truth that is either being ignored or going unaddressed. The expression also applies to an obvious problem or risk no one wants to discuss. It is based on the idea that an elephant in a room would be impossible to overlook. Some elephants can't be and should not be ignored, particularly in the church. The normal sound advice you'll get about an obvious ongoing problem is to leave it alone, let Jesus fix it, God knows all about it or just pray on it. Yes, God knows all about it, and yes, prayer is a part of the solution. However, He wants you to address the problem. Otherwise, people will leave the church and visitors will never want to come back. Paul wrote sharp letters to the established Corinthian church because the converts were slipping back into sin and not repenting. He dealt with the issues at hand for edification and not for their destruction. Some things that are allowed to go on and on, year in and year out, are damaging to the growth of the church. The Corinthians had not repented of their uncleanness, fornication and lasciviousness, tumults (confusion, agitation), whisperings, strivings, debates, backbiting etc. They were eventually made sorry by Paul's letters and repented of their sins. When is a good time to sit down and talk about obvious problems and solutions? When you are physically approached by visitors and members who say they were offended and will never return. Is there an "elephant in the room" in your church? #wisdomthekeytoengagingthemasses

Romans 14:13; 2 Corinthians 6:3; 2 Cor. 7:8; 2 Cor. 12:20-21; 2 Cor. 13:10

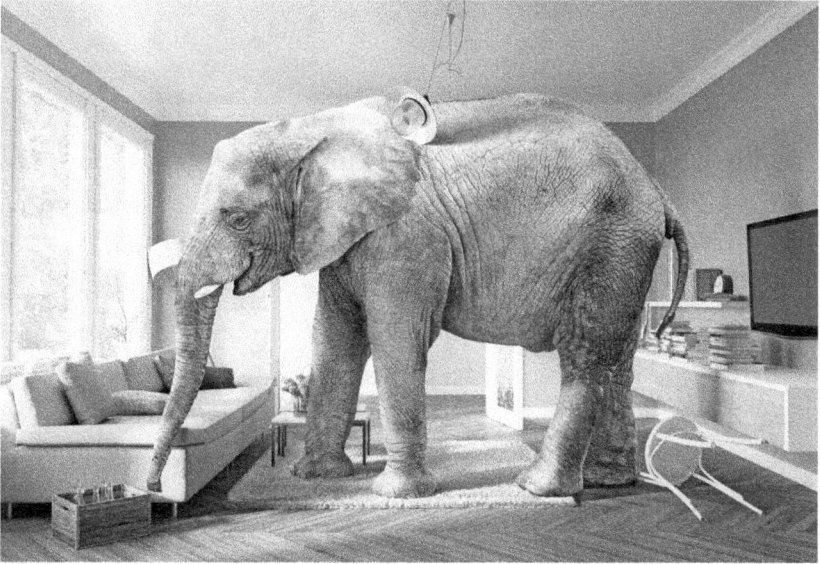

Are You Ready?

"And I saw a great white throne and Him that sat on it, from whose face the earth and the Heaven fled away, and there was found no place for them. And I saw the dead, small and great, stand before God. And, the books were opened, and another book was opened which is the Book of Life. And the dead were judged out of those things that were written in the books according to their works. And the sea gave up the dead which were in it, and Death and Hell delivered up the dead which were in them. And they were judged every man according to their works. And Death and Hell were cast into the Lake of Fire. This is the second death. And whosoever was not found written in the Book of Life was cast into the Lake of Fire."

John, the servant of Jesus Christ, was exiled to the isle of Patmos and wrote to encourage his fellow Christians as they were facing persecution in Rome. He wrote the visions that were given to him revealing those things that will come to pass.

In our earthly courts, the judge hears testimony and documented facts of the case from representing attorneys. The selected jury listens, a verdict is rendered, and the defendant is sentenced or set free as a result. "God so loved the world, that he gave His only begotten Son that whosoever believes in Him should not perish but have everlasting life." Jesus Christ is our Representative here on earth, who pleads our case to God the Father and the Judge. The documented facts are being recorded. What facts? Your works here on earth. Are you prepared to meet God? Is your name written in the Book of Life? Prepare your soul today. Give Jesus Christ your heart. Confess your sins to Him. Receive Him as your personal Savior and Representative for God. #redeemingthetime

Revelation 20:11-13; John 3:16

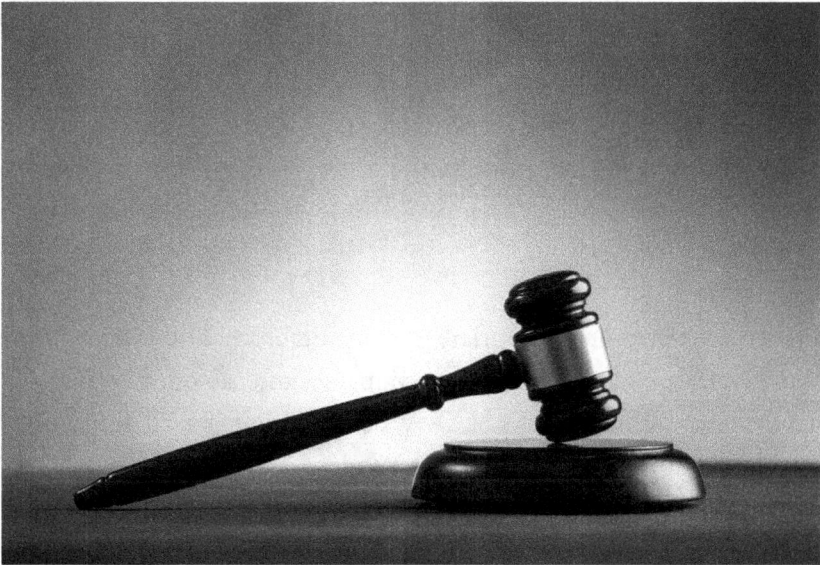

A Word Fitly Spoken

"Like apples of gold in pictures of silver" is a description given in scripture to describe the words we speak. King Solomon spoke this proverb instructing to refrain from discord, quarreling and hostility. When we think of gold and silver, we think of something that's valuable as well as pleasant to look at. When used in a positive manner, silver and gold can be the resource to provide monetary assistance and momentary happiness and pleasure. Apples are sweet and also nutritious.

When spoken in an appropriate and or suitable manner, our words can be pleasurable, healthy, sweet, valuable, and can offer assistance to the hearer. PICTURE THAT. When sharing my faith and testimony with the Leader of the Free World, I asked the Lord to give me the appropriate words. Following the example given in scripture, I received a three-paragraph, personal and timely response from the President of the United States.

I am comforted and also grateful that the word of God in a letter was chosen among many that are written on a daily basis, and that God will give the increase.

"WORDS CAN LIFT YOU UP OR WORDS CAN TEAR YOU DOWN, START A FIRE IN YOUR HEART OR PUT IT OUT."
Hawk Nelson #redeemingthetime

Proverbs 25:11; 1 Corinthians 3:7

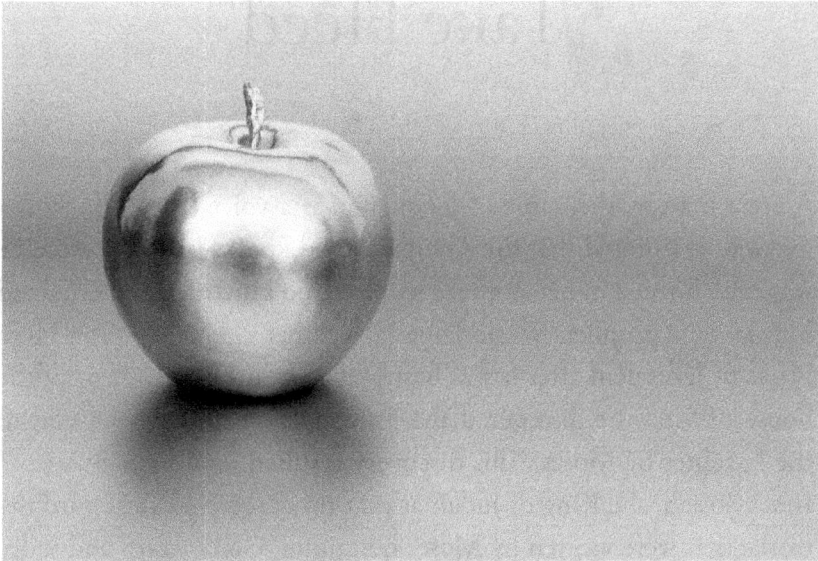

Take Heed

A great man by the name of Jeremiah was a voice especially chosen by God. It is noted that the Almighty God knew Jeremiah before he was even formed in his mother's womb. God sanctified and ordained him to be a prophet. While Jeremiah's father (Hilkiah) was a High Priest in Jerusalem after it was besieged and during the repair of the house of God, he discovered the lost book of the Laws written to the Israelites by Moses. This discovery resulted in the repentance of Israel. Josiah, the King of Judah at that time, received and heard the words that were written by Moses describing God's wrath and judgments toward his people for not keeping the word of the Lord.

These words were confirmed by a prophetess (Huldah) warning the King, revealing that evil would come upon the inhabitants because they were still provoking God with their wickedness. But because of his tender heart and his humble spirit, he would not see all the evil he would bring and would rest in peace with his fathers. Before he passed, King Josiah took away all the abominations out of all the countries that pertained to the children of Israel and made all that were present in Israel serve the Lord their God. Jeremiah told God because he was a child, he could not speak to the people to warn them. But God touched his mouth and said, "I have put my words in your mouth. Be not afraid of their faces." It was at this time that Jeremiah was prepared to plead with and warn the inhabitants of the land (the Israelites) to turn back to God.

This short history reveals the heart of the Almighty God and his multitudes of mercies. God regarded the affliction of his people even though their sins brought him to the point of "abhorring his inheritance." He remembered his covenant with them. Hearing their cries, he made their enemies and capturers pity them as well as reversing his judgments upon them. We, the Gentiles, the non-Jews, the body of Christ, are grafted into the vines of God's chosen people. If God spared not his natural branches from severe judgment, we the church need to take heed least we are not spared.

Sin has not ceased in the synagogues, cathedrals, churches, and anywhere where God's name is established. Technology has made it possible to spread the gospel of Jesus Christ in every direction. But technology has also made it possible to stream live the sins and failures of those who were trusted with the gifts of God and his word. The children of Israel and Judah turned to false idols and other gods, causing their sons and daughters to die in sacrifice by fire. Today our children are subjected to pedophiles in the pulpit and in the confession booth. They are being sold into sex slavery and aborted in the womb, supported by people in high places. God warned his people, saying, "Though you wash with soap and other hygiene products, your iniquity and sin is marked before me." Today, money can buy any treatment to enhance the hygiene and wellbeing of the outward appearance but cannot cover the vile affections woven into every level of society in disobedience to God's word.

We, the people of God, are not to be comfortable with the normalization of sin against the word of God. God looked for at least one person who would say, "This is not right" in the cities of Sodom and Gomorrah, where men and women were burned in lust toward the same sex. Both cities were destroyed by fire and brimstone. Jeremiah suffered great persecution for warning against sin among the people of God. He was buried in mud but rescued. There is no record of his death. Whatever church or place of worship you are in today, don't frustrate the Grace of God. Repent and be the light God has chosen you to be. #redeemingthetime

Jeremiah Chapter 1; 2 Chronicles 34:14-22

Blessings In Disguise

I was in the 12th grade working overtime on my high school year-book during the Cuban Missile Crisis. While standing by the classroom window, I noticed the sunset displaying very vivid orange and red clouds, creating a beautiful sight, only to be spoiled by my next thought. *When is it going to happen? Is this what a nuclear holocaust looks like?* I was one among many who were daily in fear of a bad outcome. I would get a sick feeling in the pit of my stomach each time the news was broadcast on every channel. These were feelings that I wished would go away. I didn't know the Lord at the age of 18, therefore I could not be comforted in knowing that God was in control of the situation and that my name was written in the Lamb's book of life.

Eventually, the crisis was resolved, tensions relieved, and many promises broken to God. However, I can't recall doing anything to make my life right with God during that time. I thought I was okay because I attended church every Sunday and served on the Usher Board. Five years later I met Jesus Christ at the altar while repenting of my sins. I was in a crisis of my own and desperate for God. He heard me and saved me. Our trials in life are blessings in disguise that bring us to where God wants us to be.

God will hear you. He knows your heart and all of your fears. Trust him with your life. There are many things happening all over that warrant our attention. Nevertheless, God can give you the peace that passes all understanding, that the world could never give. Many have already decided to dismiss the Almighty God and his plan for man. God is a gentleman and will not violate your right of choice. Come out from among them and trust God with your life. Receive God's love gift to the world, Jesus Christ as your personal savior. "For God so loved the world that he gave his only begotten son that whosoever believes in him should not perish but have everlasting life." #redeemingthetime

John 3:16; 2 Corinthians 6:17; Joshua 24:15; Revelation 21:27; Romans 10:13

God Bless The Children

Praying for the children. Too much tragedy all over the world, particularly concerning the children. Father, watch over them to and from school. Have mercy on those who seek to bring them harm. Stop the plan of the enemy to destroy their dreams, their goals, their lives. Move them out of situations where parents and guardians care more about themselves, which places them in dangerous situations. Continue to send good Samaritans to feed them, clothe them, and shelter them. Have mercy, oh God. You said in your Word that your mercy endures forever. Let your hand of mercy be extended here and all over the world. Today is a day of tears for the children. Hear my cry, Father, in the name of Jesus. GOD BLESS THE CHILDREN.

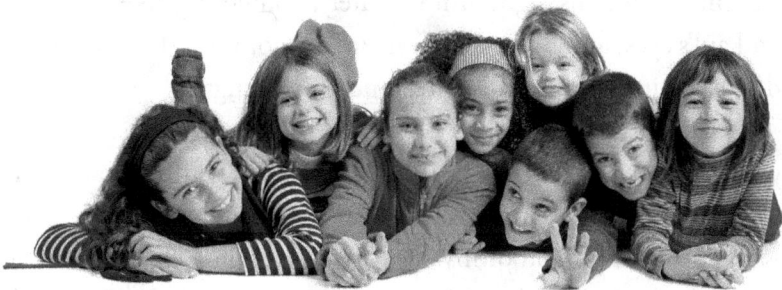

Once I Was Blind

At the end of a conversation I was having with my son, I told him I was praying that the Lord would remove the scales from his eyes. About a week later he asked, "What did you mean by remove the scales from my eyes?" We were in a discussion about the importance of receiving Jesus Christ as the Redeemer and Savior of the soul. In response, my son urged me to explore other religions via various history books in challenge to the divine status of Jesus Christ.

Paul, a man chosen by God, met the Lord via a flashing light that shined from Heaven. Paul was responsible for the murder of many Christians who were cast into prison for calling upon the name of the Lord. At this encounter, Paul became a chosen instrument to proclaim God's name to the Gentiles and their kings and to the people of Israel. God blinded his eyes for three days until he sent a man that he might receive his sight. Immediately, something like scales fell from Paul's eyes, and he could see again. He got up and was baptized, and after taking some food, he regained his strength.

My first encounter with the Lord came at the church altar one Saturday night in the early 70s. I sang and praised the Lord for saving me after repenting of all of my sins. I was rejoicing all the way from the church to the number 10 bus stop across from the Red-Light district the Block. A man walked by and asked, "How's tricks?" and kept on walking. I responded, "Fine!" thinking he said how's church.

I realized later that God had this little newborn baby all hedged up and protected on the Block. The next morning, I woke up to everything appearing brand new. The trees, flowers and sky seemed more beautiful than ever. The scales had been removed from my eyes.

Father, move on us the Body of Christ throughout the world to focus on the Commission of capturing the lost, discarded and underserved. At each encounter, let our light shine so bright that the scales would fall from their eyes, unveiling your glory and unending love. #redeemingthetime

Acts Chapter 9

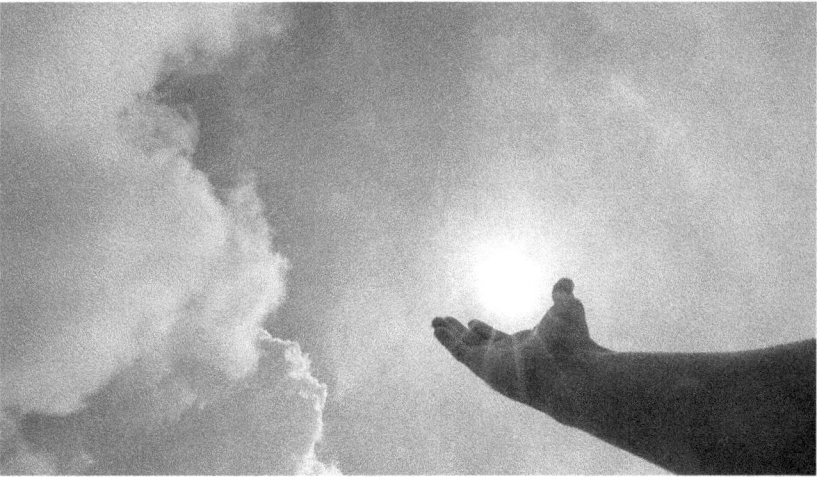

Holy Ground

My little mama took her shoes off in church yesterday. I asked why. Her response: "This is Holy ground."

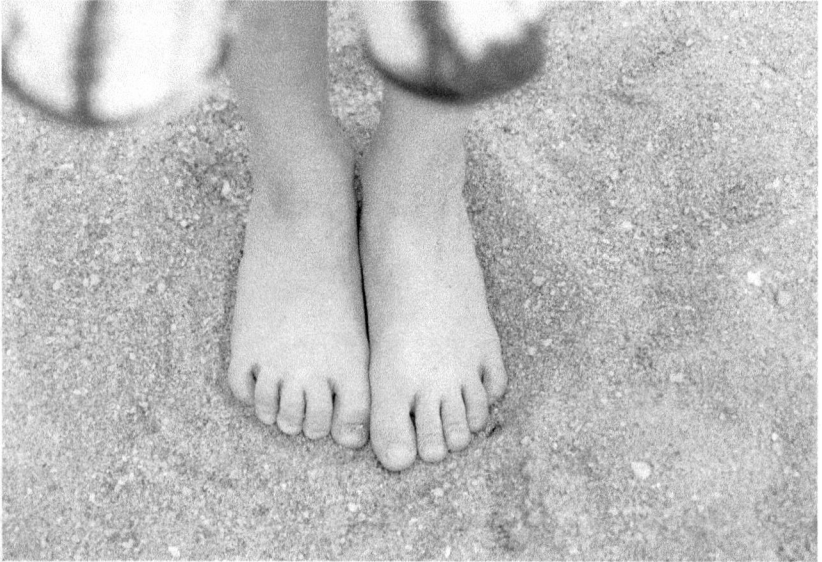

Honor

The magnificent honor and home-going celebration of President George H. W. Bush was truly an event fit for a President. I laughed, cried and engaged every moment, especially the orchestra and classical music, along with all who were in attendance. I can't help but think that God was watching the entire service, focusing on the words uttered in eulogy from the heart of President Bush.

And I believe that leaders and people worldwide were able to hear and be inspired. "Never be defined by failure." "Serving others enriches the givers' soul." Most importantly was the quote "Hate corrodes the container it's carried in." President George H. W. Bush has gone on to meet with the judge of the world to give an account for his deeds done while here on earth. His inspiring words will remain and live in the hearts of his family and go down in history to affect future leaders and generations to come.

Let us not discount what God can do in the hearts of an unregenerated world to draw them closer to Him. #redeemingthetime

(Image of a flag draped coffin)

Camp Meeting

LAWD HAVE MERCY!! Camp Meeting 2017 was off the chain. Wish you could have been there. Camp Meeting is just what it says. Meet to "camp out" in the presence of the Lord. Praying and seeking the Lord at a designated time for a visitation from on high is the yearly "Great Expectation" of the Saints of God. It is a special time to push the plate back, repent, commit, recommit, renew, sing, praise, and dance before the Lord. It is a time to be refreshed by the Anointed Word of God via his Chosen and Anointed vessels. It is a time to get desperate to please the Almighty God and be blessed.

King David danced with all his might in the presence of the Lord. The people, along with David, shouted and played on all manner of instruments, including trumpets, cymbals, harps, drums cornets and more, while in God's presence.

I couldn't get enough of being under the cloud of anointing and blessings in this Camp Meeting 2017. So what's next? The designated time of expectation has passed. Our cups are filled and overflowing. Our hearts have been mended in love toward one another. A hunger for righteousness is present in the house of God. A focus on unity and love is evident. God has saved us and called us to a Holy Calling, and He is able to keep that which we have committed unto Him for his purpose. Somebody needs the Lord. Now is the time to lift up Jesus with that power and anointing received from God. The world will not be able to gain-say or resist the Gospel (Good news). As mentioned in the morning message via Pastor Sharon Hardy Knotts, "There is something in the heart of God He enjoys as his people chase after him." Keep seeking the Lord and please Him throughout the year. #redeemingthetime

2 Samuel 6:5,14; Matthew 5:6; 2 Timothy 1:9; Luke 21:15

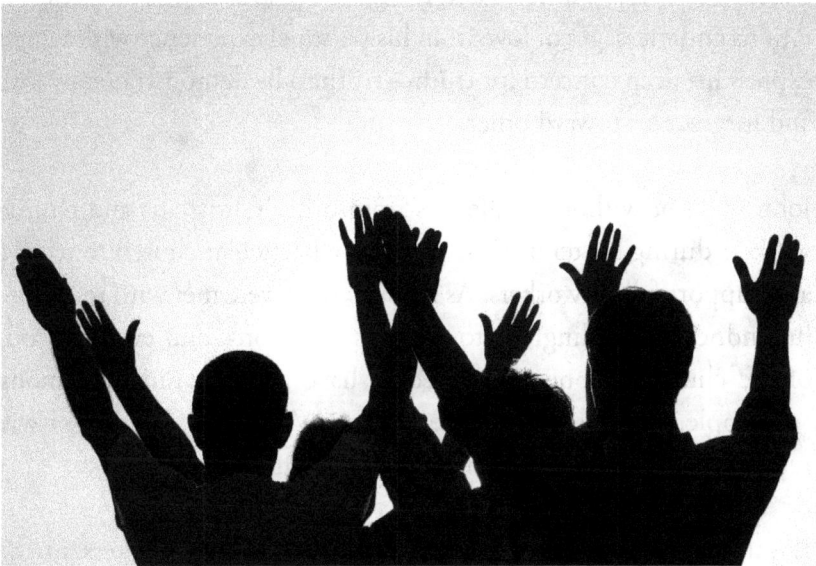

Challenge

John, known as The Beloved Apostle, is believed to have been the author of the Book of John and the three Epistles of John. His exhortations and messages of love from his personal experience with Christ express his deep concern for truth—truth to be demonstrated by love and forgiveness toward others.

John was not without challenges from other Christians and church workers during his tenure. He wrote to a particular church to receive and support fellow workers. As a result, they were met with rejection, unkindness, unwillingness to accept suggestions, and even cast out of the church by one who loved to have the preeminence among the people. The beloved apostle wrote, "Wherefore if I come, I will remember the deeds which he doeth." (3 John 1:10, KJV)

Loyal brothers and sisters deserve support. Fellow workers in the Lord should be received with joy. Consistent negative overtones and undisciplined spirits hinder the work of God. No doubt, John had his work cut out for him in challenging unruly behavior in the name of Christian fellowship. Be the challenge. Work together in love. #redeemingthetime

Book of St. John; The First Epistle of John; The Second Epistle of John; The Third Epistle of John

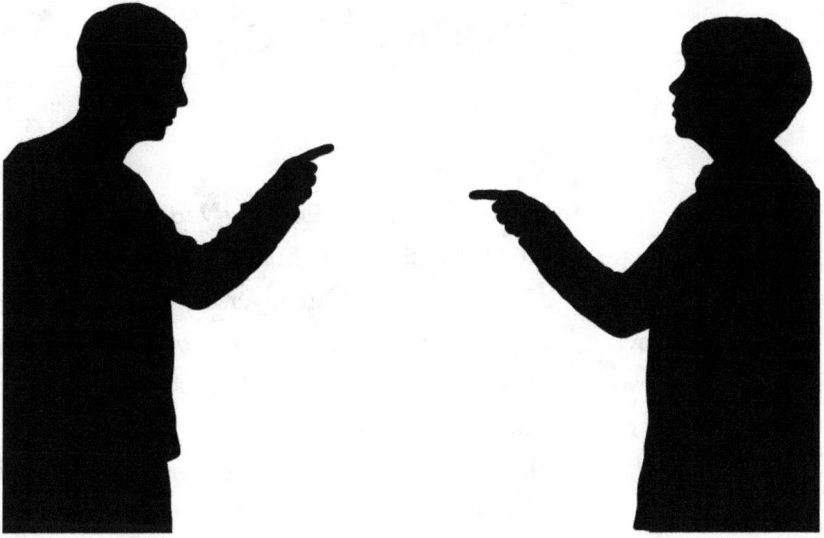

Checkmate!

Chess is an awesome game of strategy. Blocking your opponent to reach the ultimate goal requires skill, thought and knowledge of each individual chess piece and its function. Our adversary Satan is having a field day moving his pieces around on his chessboard of evil. He knows exactly who to use in accomplishing his purpose to promote discord, hate, tragedy, injustice and outright sin against the Almighty God. It would appear that his most hellish demons unleashed in the world are winning the game.

NOT SO FAST! God has an army that is breaking the chains of evil every day. God has people in strategic places all over the world that have not bowed down to sin and depravity. He knows where Satan's seat is located. There are those among you who are wide awake, constant in prayer and fasting, active against injustice and pushing back the darkness and evil gripping this planet.

Let's remain steadfast in the work of the Lord. Don't give in to the adversary as one of his pawns that move the world's inhabitants away from God. In Satan's strategy, he knows we will not commit the obvious sins. But he easily works through pride, over- and self-indulgence, unforgiveness, biases, self-righteousness, and improper responses for all the world to see. These put us in an AWOL status in God's army of trusted soldiers. Let us consider the lines and verses of the gospel lyrics we've been singing down through the years and apply them.

Break Every Chain. Onward Christian Soldiers Marching On To War. Jesus Keep Me Near The Cross. I Give Myself Away. #redeemingthetime

1 Peter 5:8; John 10:10; 2 Timothy 2::4; Ephesians 6::12; Proverbs 25:26

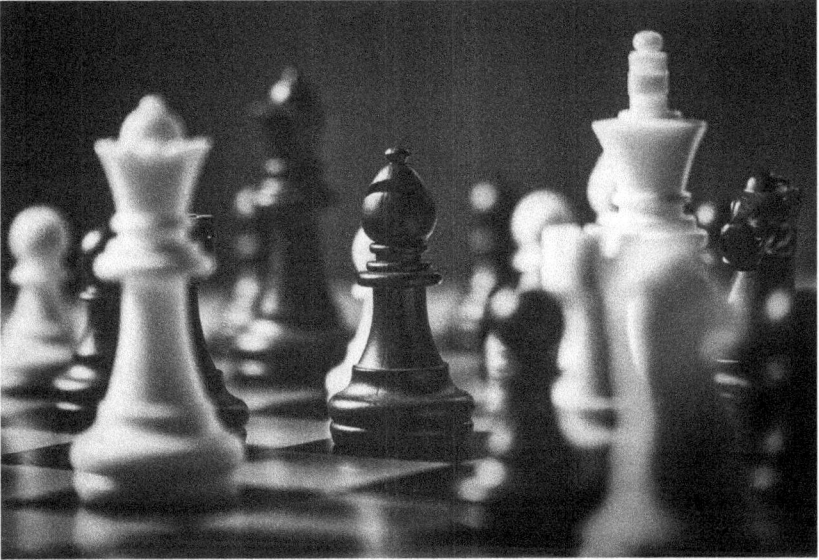

Choose Prayerfully

In every facet of our lives, we are faced with choices. These may include what we eat, where we live, the friends we choose, the schools we decide to attend, or the jobs we select to meet our daily needs. In so many words, we form our destiny. And the destiny we choose determines how our lives "play out." God is a gentleman and will not violate our right of choice, simply because he wants us to choose to love Him. (Joshua 24:14-15).

Whatever the circumstances, it is a place of your choosing. If your choices place you on the other side of God's plan for your life, God knows your heart. He will urge you by His Holy Spirit to obey His Word, but ultimately leave the decision up to you. He sets before you life and death (Deuteronomy 30:15). You are not alone in your struggle to please God. We have an adversary, the devil, who desires to move us far from God. However, he was already defeated on the Cross of Calvary (1 John 3:8). Our failures are just steppingstones to victory! Do not dwell on the failure but continue in the battle to please God.

Repent, get up and keep moving forward. Surround yourself with Christian friends. Attend church if possible. Talk to God every day and let Him know you are trying. He knows all about you. Most importantly, study the Word of God for instruction and inspiration (2 Timothy 2:15). Obedience is better than sacrifice (1 Samuel

15:22). God acts upon a simple prayer of repentance, truly from the heart: "Dear Lord. Be merciful to me, a sinner. Wash me in Your blood. Forgive me of all of my sins. Cleanse me from all unrighteousness. I receive You as my Savior and confess You as my Lord." God will forever change your life!

Dear Lord, touch our lives with Your tenderness and love. Lead, guide and direct us into Your perfect Will. Reveal Your plan for our lives as we seek You daily. Bring about new circumstances and opportunities in our lives that move us toward You.

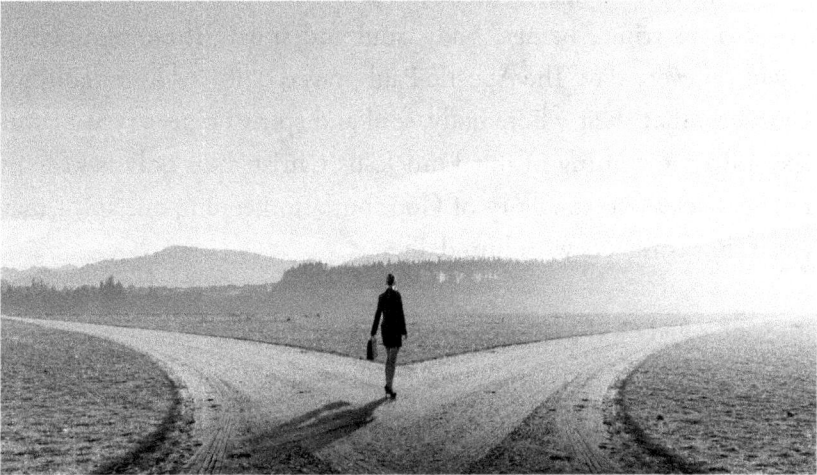

Cleansing

A good shower or bath involves getting at all the right spots to assure cleanliness. Continuing to miss them or even skipping on a regular basis brings undesired results. Odor, itching, loss of friends, just to name a few, are the results that make the body cry out for a thorough cleansing. I thank God that in all his wisdom, he formed and fashioned us as triune beings, body, soul and spirit. These require our attention every day. The Apostle Paul prayed daily for his established churches, that their whole body, soul and spirit be preserved blameless unto the coming of our Lord Jesus Christ. Not only is keeping the body clean to the glory of God, but also keeping our spirit man clean that connects with him daily.

Today I asked God in prayer to remove those things deep in my heart that may produce an undesired result. I also asked him to remove those things received in my spirit that I chose to reject but that were still causing disgust, frustration and anger, particularly during times of testing. Keeping "stuff" brewing in the spirit man may cause you to say the wrong thing at the wrong time to the wrong people, resulting in a "snowball" of events. "I'm turning it over to you Lord. My spirit needs a good bath." We can win the victory over sin, but an ongoing filthy spirit can cause life-long effects to others. I ministered to my 95-year-old neighbor before she passed and was able to help her overcome the effects of a troubling incident that happened many years ago. She was crying and couldn't understand why after so many years of being in the same church, her opponent could not forgive her of a wrong committed. We prayed together, asking God to bring healing to her spirit as well as healing to the opponent. She had carried that pain all those years. Unwillingness to forgive is an undesired result that can create a "snowball" of events.

How we affect others in our daily conversation and walk in the Lord is of utmost importance to God. #keepingitreal

1 Thessalonians 5:23; 2 Corinthians 7:1; 2 Corinthians 3:2-5; Philippians 2:3-6

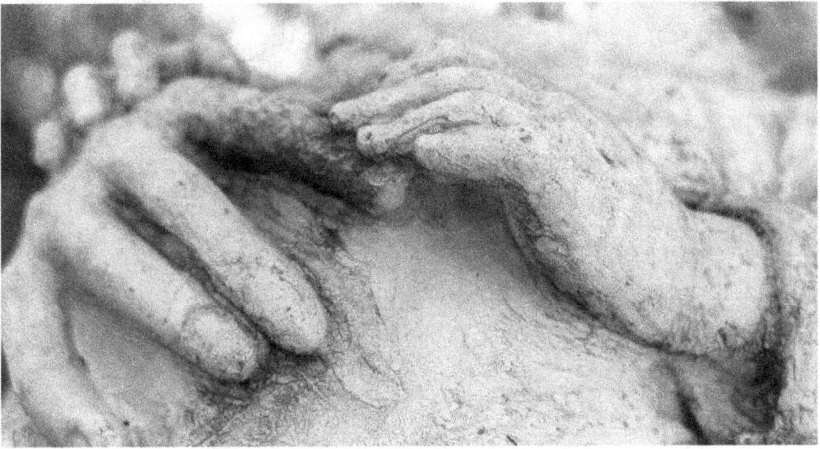

Climate - Prayer

It was a glorious day in 1963 when my sister and I paid 25 cents to board a yellow school bus headed for Washington, D. C. A Godly man with a powerful voice, chosen of God, mobilized African Americans from every corner of this nation for a "March on Washington." Reverend Dr. Martin Luther King Jr. was the voice for his people to address the nation's need for change within a racist society. We had a ring-sized seat at the reflecting pool to hear the many voices speaking on the issues. We were teenagers at the time and our father was strictly opposed to us participating, fearful that "Mr. Charlie" would get us. With three decades between him and slavery, his mindset was to keep quiet and not make any waves. That generation's "Mr. Charlie" was the white man. Our ancestors were severely oppressed mentally as well as physically, passing down the oral tradition from one generation to the next.

Our mother intervened and we were able to take the trip to Washington, D. C. Sitting at the reflecting pool, listening to all the voices, seeing all the people from various religious and ethnic backgrounds, all in support of the cause, was a moment in time never to be forgotten. Then came Reverend Martin Luther King Jr.'s "I Have a Dream" speech. My spirit was lifted and filled with hope for change. We returned to our communities to mobilize, march, sit-in and do what was necessary to peacefully effect change. The "Dream" happened, overriding decades of laws that enforced racial segregation and laws placed to prevent black men from casting a ballot. Jim

Crow laws were intended to remove political and economic gains and limit the freedom and opportunity of people of color.

Then it happened. Reverend Dr. Martin Luther King Jr. was murdered April 4, 1968. The voice God chose to bring awareness to injustice and bring about political and economic gain for blacks was gunned down and murdered. What followed? Another black man, a powerful black man, was murdered. One hundred and twenty-three cities in the U. S. marched in protest over the murder of Reverend Dr. Martin Luther King Jr. Maryland's Governor Agnew called for the State Police and National Guard to manage the riots that were also triggered by the murder. Armed troops were requested and deployed to Baltimore and other areas. All transit bus service was suspended. A curfew was enforced. Some had to walk to work. At the end of our work shift, each employee was escorted to their home via a charter bus and an armed soldier.

Political and economic change produced by people of color disturbs and exposes the evil still among us, lurking and interwoven in places we wouldn't expect. Many have given their lives for justice in this country. Despite resistance, the platform for change will continue. Let us continue to pray that this evil will be rooted out forever.

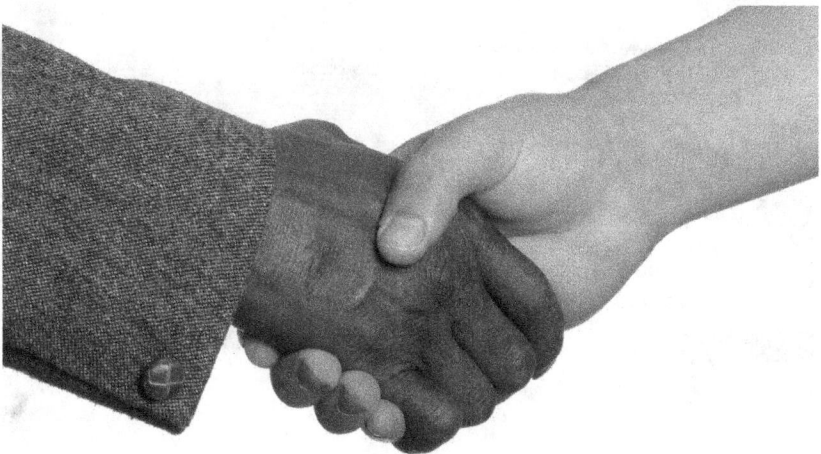

Come Boldly

Joab fled to the tabernacle and grabbed hold of the horns of the Altar of Sacrifice, expecting to die there (1 Kings 2:28-29). Now, in our time of trouble we can come to the throne of GRACE, making our petitions known unto God through His love gift Jesus Christ. His Mercy endures forever!

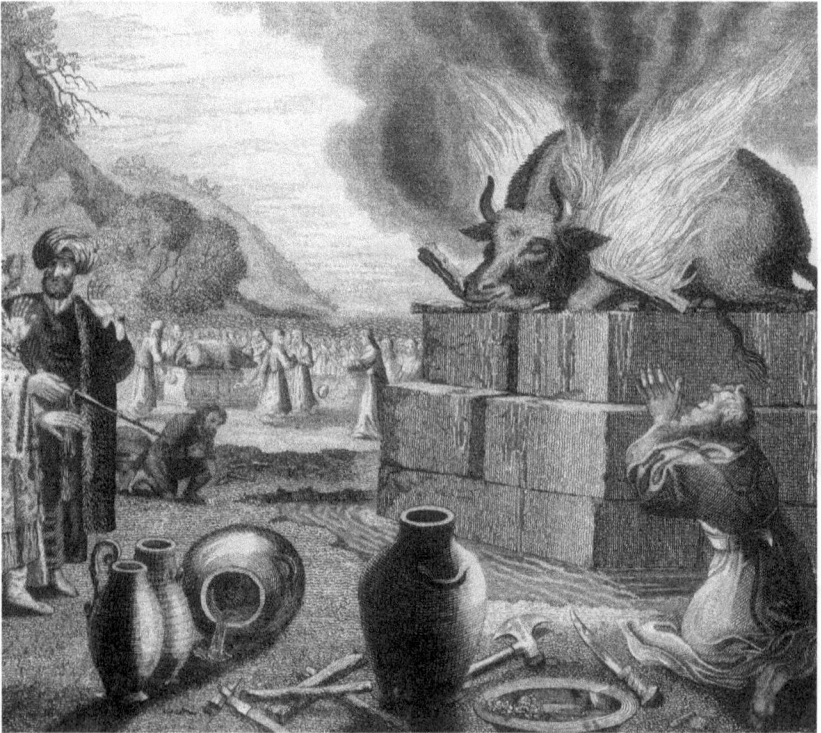

The Creator's Example

I responded to a post shared by one of my millennial relatives relating to his concerns about climate change. It was titled "GENTLE REMINDER THAT THE EARTH IS DYING AND WE ARE TOO." Pictures were also posted of the same, to bring to mind the devastating results including the abundance of CO_2 in the atmosphere, large penguin colonies disappearing, endangered animals facing extinction and expert testimonies and warnings by scientists to the earth's inhabitants of impending doom. The massive responses to this post were divisive and very evident that many are in fear of what the future holds.

The Bible reminds us all that death is imminent. Even the very creatures God created are patiently waiting for their change, along with the children of God, for the redemption of the body from the bondage of corruption. I was then asked, "Do you feel like in this case we should wait it out or let God fix it?" In response:

God has given us the tools, along with divine knowledge, to manage his creations from the very beginning of time, as well as to prepare for our transition. Unfortunately, greed and power have gotten into the mix over the eons of time, clouding the minds of those who can make a difference, particularly with climate change. The condition of our existence is in direct relationship to the choices we make and the resulting outcomes. Yes, God could intervene and fix it all. However, he will not violate our right to choose right from wrong. Further reading into his plan via the Bible points out his desire for willing obedience to him in love. We have an adversary whose job is to influence many to stray from God's divine plan for all inhabitants of the earth. Therefore, every evil deed, atrocity, destruction, mayhem, etc., is blamed on the Almighty Creator, when in fact it's all a direct result of choices made in opposition to God's divine plan for man. There you have it. The fight between good and evil will exist until God says enough is enough. He is not willing that any should perish, die, or be destroyed, but that all should come to the knowledge of the truth. Dying is not the end. Jesus Christ is the Hope of Glory. #redeemingthetime

John 3:16; 2 Peter 3:9; 1Timothy 2:4; Romans 8:19-25; Matthew 7:13-14; John 14:23; Colossians 1:27

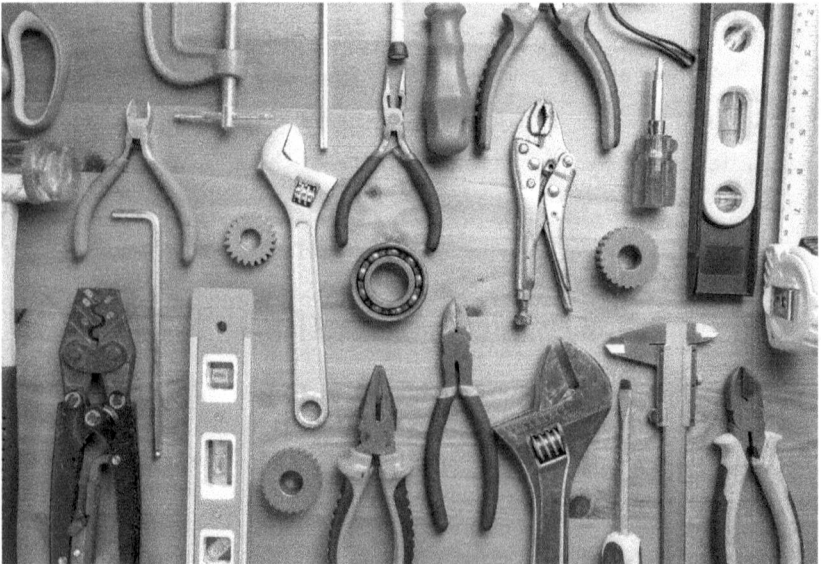

Don't Bow

Saints of God, Christians, and fellow workers in Christ, draw closer to the Savior and remain steadfast in what you have been called to do. Continue in fasting, prayers, good works, and brotherly kindness.

Paul in his letters to the churches often encouraged his fellow workers, who were met with many obstacles and barriers for Christ. God's mercy is enduring. Continue to seek and save those who are lost. God has a number who are not asleep and have not "bowed their knee to Baal." #redeemingthetime

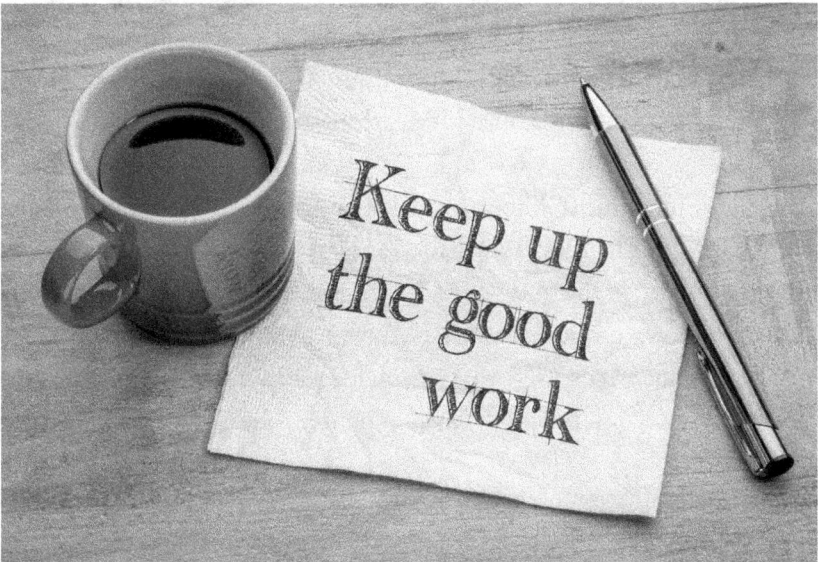

Do The Right Thing

David, the giant killer, grew to be a man who loved God. As the scripture says, he was a man after God's own heart. Through his own life experiences, David found God to be merciful, compassionate and true to his word. He asked a question: "Who shall abide in God's tabernacle and who shall dwell in his holy hill?"

The events that took place in David's life allowed him to pen his responses to these questions. He learned that he must walk upright, do the right things before God and speak the truth in his heart. At one point in his life, David plotted and schemed to get another man's wife. He committed adultery and arranged the death of the husband of his mistress. No doubt he used his power to cause the death of an innocent man. The instruction went out to place the husband on the front lines of battle to assure his death in the same.

The messenger most likely reaped a military or monetary benefit from carrying out David's instructions. David explained in his writings that if you want to dwell in God's tabernacle and in his holy hill don't use your money for evil purposes. Money becomes the root of all evil when it is used to manipulate evil schemes and cause the death of innocent people. David repented with tears and received God's mercy.

We can learn a lot through our own unconfessed sins and short-comings and have our relationships restored with God. And in the process, someone else can be blessed and restored because we learned like David to repent and speak the truth in our hearts. God honors those who fear him and want to do the right thing. Fall upon God's mercy today. Repent and give him your heart. "For God so loved the world that he gave his only begotten Son Jesus Christ, that who-soever believes in him should not perish but have everlasting life." #redeemingthetime

Acts 13:22; Psalm 15; Samuel Chapter 11; John 3:16

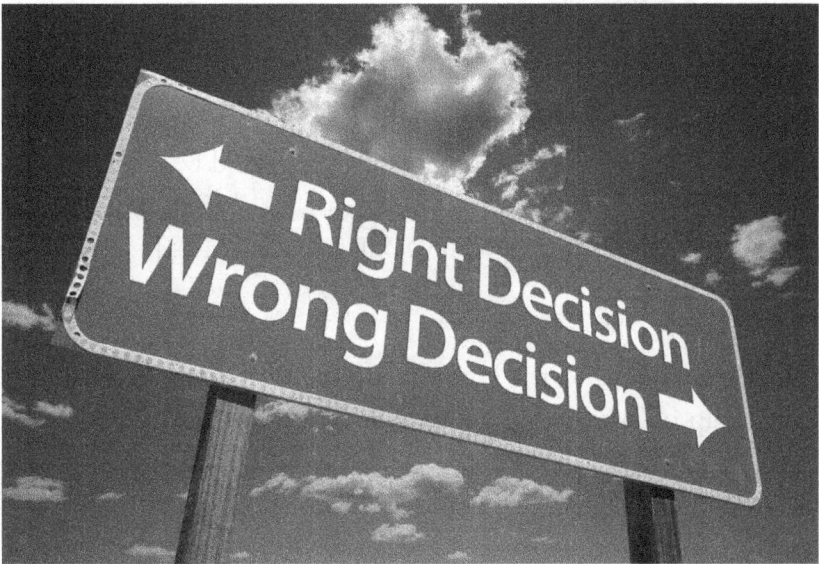

On Eagle's Wings

I saw a video of an eagle flying high in the sky. A camera had been strategically placed on the bird to give the viewer an "eagle's experience while in flight." It was an awesome sight, putting me "at one with nature" in real-time. Our Everlasting God, the Lord, the Creator of this beautiful creature gives it its strength, swiftness, and powerful wings to soar high in the sky.

Symbolic of the eagle's strength, God said he carried his people on eagle's wings and brought them out of Egypt. In times of severe testing and trials, we can look to God's promises and be encouraged to remain faithful in the battle. God doesn't faint or get weary. He gives power to the faint, and to them who have no might he increases their strength. Been there?

"They that wait upon the Lord shall renew their strength. They shall mount up on wings of an eagle. They shall run and not be weary. They shall walk and not faint." "And let us not be weary in well doing for in due season we shall reap, if we faint not." #redeemingthetime

Exodus 19:4; Isaiah 40:28-31; Galatians 6:9

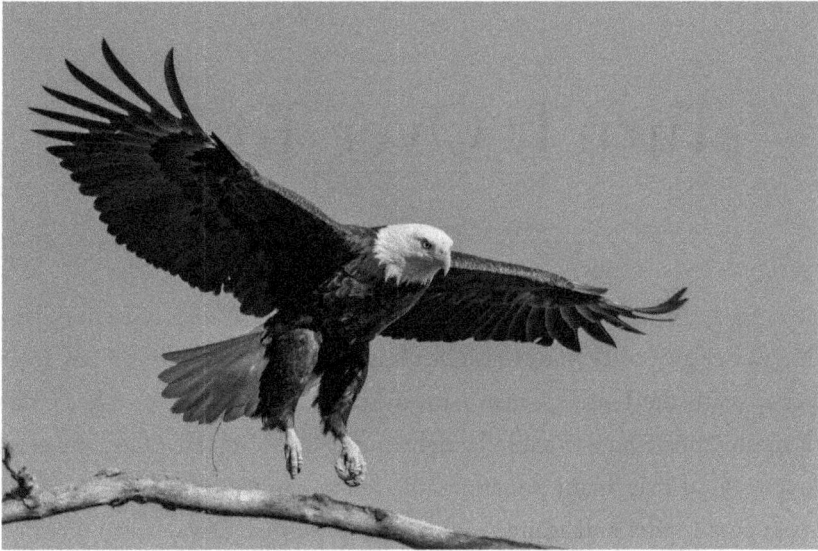

Turn It Over To God

Let the Lord fight your battles. "Dearly beloved, avenge not yourselves, but rather give place unto wrath: for it is written, Vengeance is mine; I will repay, saith the Lord." A man named David in the Bible was after God's heart and one who wanted to be righteous before Him. He called and cried out to God over many situations that were happening in his life. There were people after and against him for many reasons. David called them his enemies who fought against and persecuted him.

In my earlier years, I can think of one person who I called an enemy who would not be satisfied until they had me in their grip for a beat down. It came to a head when they decided to confront me at the community library. Unlike David, I didn't know anything about crying out to God for help to fight against my enemies. Therefore, the event became somewhat of an entertainment to those looking on. The cat fight was on, ending with bruises and a flattened ego.

David cried unto God asking Him to deal with those people who set out to hurt him. He specifically outlined what he wanted God to do concerning his enemies. In his prayer, he asked God to let the angel of the Lord persecute them, let their way be dark and slippery, pull out his spear and stop them in their way and let them be turned back and brought to confusion. God knows how to stop the plan of our adversary Satan and the vessels he uses against us. Now that we know the Lord, we can trust him and let him fight all of our battles and keep our "enemies at bay".

#redeemingthetime Romans 12:19 - Psalm 35

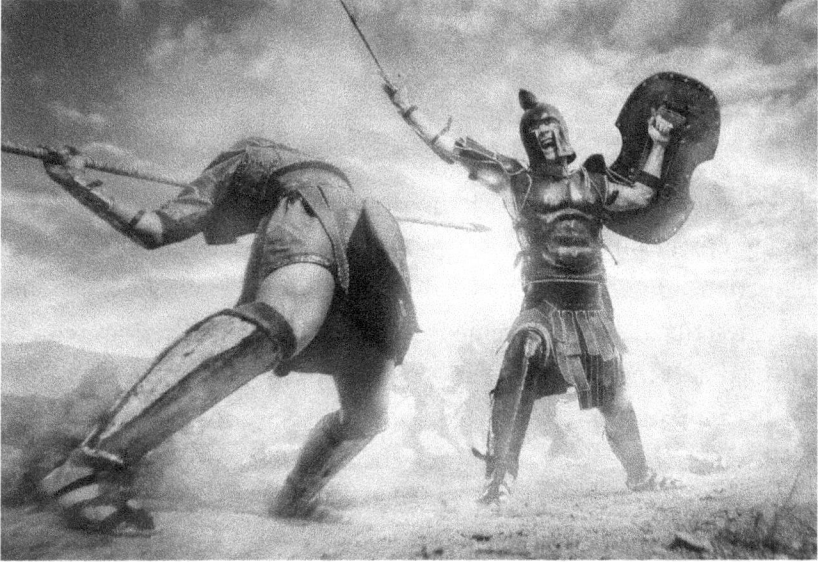

Fight The Good Fight

To tell the Good News that Jesus saves and to share the Word of God about His healing power is a most important Commission for the Christian. One day in this Christian walk, there was an experience so indescribable that movement or breathing caused serious pain. It affected speech, movement and every activity that involved mobility. It came at a time when much help was needed to bring forth a soul-winning event in the church. In the process, the Word of God came as FOOD and LIFE to meet the need. He took my infirmities and bore my sicknesses...He by whose stripes we were healed bore my sins on the tree, that I, being dead to sin, should live unto righteousness (Matthew 8:17; 1 Peter 2:24).

Living God's Word has taught patience through trials, appreciation for His exceedingly great and precious promises, and compassion for others. I've learned how to stand firm and unmovable on His Word, and most importantly, TRUST IN GODS' WORD.

1 Peter 4:12-13, KJV... "Beloved, think it not strange concerning the fiery trial, which is to try you, as though some strange thing happened unto you. But rejoice, inasmuch as ye are partakers of Christ's sufferings, that, when His glory shall be revealed, ye may be glad also with exceeding joy."

TO ALL WHO ARE FIGHTING THE GOOD FIGHT OF FAITH.

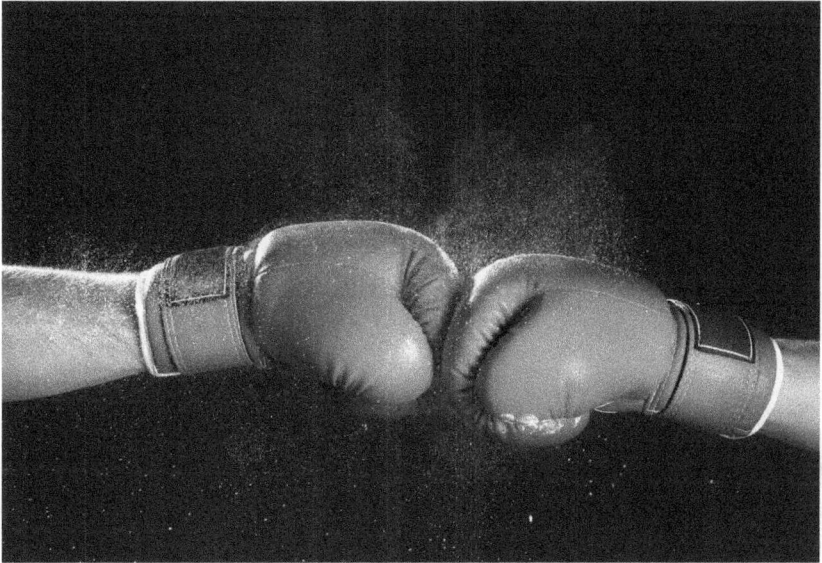

Forgive

Sometimes when we are hurt, we resort to catchy phrases and certain scriptures to fit the one(s) who brought the offense. And getting others to agree borders on discord and only offers temporary relief from the pain on the inside. FORGIVE, and turn it over to Jesus and be FREE. #redeemingthetime

Matthew 6:14

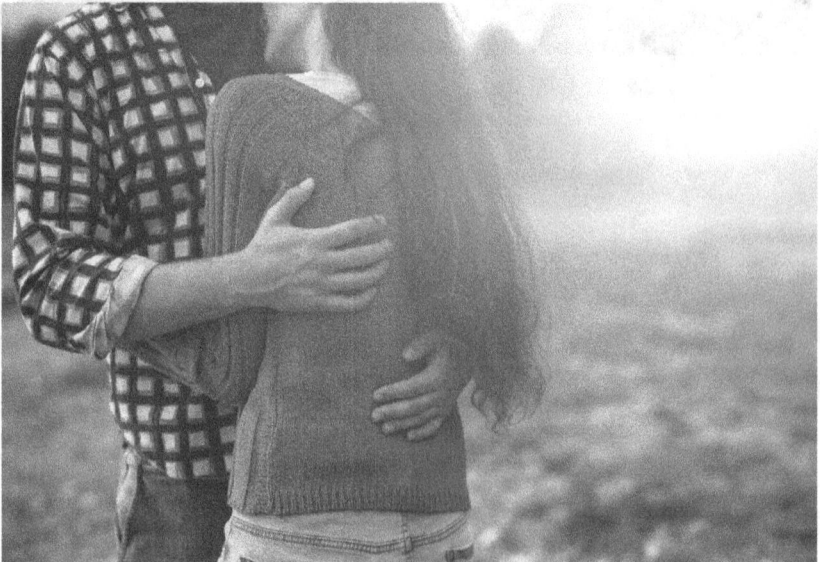

Get Back Satan!

"Get back Satan" is one of many favorite gospel songs of encouragement to the child of God experiencing the trials of life. And we know that a lot of those trials stem from our adversary Satan to bring discouragement, and loss of hope. Yesterday, after spending four days in the hospital, I returned home oppressed by Satan concerning my health. He was working hard with his suggestions to weaken my faith and trust in God. I could barely get my prayer through without telling him to shut up several times. He can be ruthless in his attack when it comes to discrediting God while counting on you to forget the Word of God and all the accounts mentioned of God's wonderful works.

I got up from prayer, knowing God again heard not only my spoken words but those feelings pressed deeply in my spirit, generating the necessary tears in that moment. "Whenever the devil tries to turn you around, just keep on praying and stand your ground!" "Praise His (God's) name and hold your head up high!" These lyrics as well as others expressed in song bring encouragement in the many "tight spots" of a Christian.

Moments after this experience, I received a text out of nowhere that read: "I will get you through this. God." This word of encouragement and note from God came at the right time via the vessel God chose to use. When Satan tries to make you feel you are alone in your trials, rebuke him and tell him to shut up. Our God is mindful of everything we go through and encounter while on this Christian experience. I WON'T GIVE UP OR GIVE IN. Trust God with your life. #redeemingthetime

1 Corinthians 10:13; Jude 1:9; Proverbs 30:5; Hebrews 11:1; 1 Corinthians 16:13

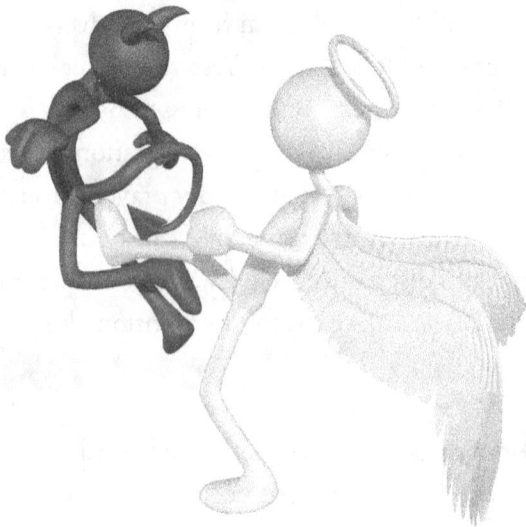

Glory From Heaven

At that place where the windows of Heaven are opened once again, God is listening. As his presence is all around, many names are going forth to his throne room. I can feel when his heart is touched because the tears won't stop flowing, particularly for those who don't have anyone to call their name out in prayer. I am at that place once again where my words can't express all that my heart wants to pour out. That's when the anointing bows me down to release the deep utterances that only God understands. That's when my entire being is projected into another realm called the Secret Place.

That's when you know that you know God is real and he hears and answers every cry from his people. When the power and anointing of God grips you so gently you know that your prayer is making a difference and that God is moving. My body feels like I just stepped out of a fresh shower draped by warm towels, and the desire for food has become a distant memory.

Let the Lord bless you today with a touch from Heaven. 2 Chronicles 7:14

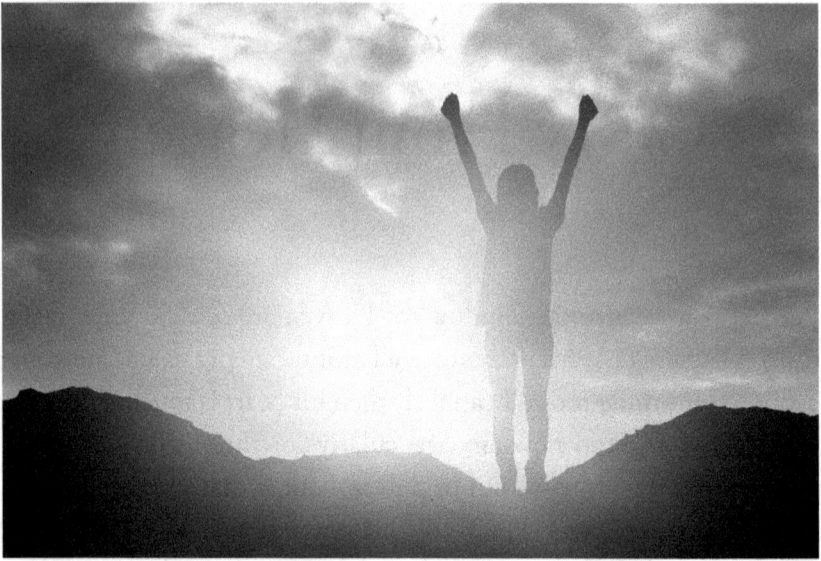

Glory In His Presence

Yesterday was a beautiful day of spiritual blessings as the Lord visited us with His sweet anointing in the praise service. His cloud of love rested over the congregation as the choir lifted Him up in song. New faces were seen wiping tears from their eyes as the Lord Himself knocked on the doors of their hearts. It was that kind of anointing that assures everything is going to be all right in the midst of troubles. The hearts were truly open to receive his love. Being in His presence was ever so sweet, etching the memory of His goodness to pass on to future generations. The effectual fervent prayers of the righteous are a help and advantage in drawing souls to the church as well as welcoming the Holy Spirit to the sanctuary each and every time the church doors are open.

I'm reminded of my initial conversion with the Lord. Although the message coming forth convicted me of my sinful condition, I couldn't help but notice and feel the love surrounding me. That anointing (the presence and power of God) that I knew nothing about at the time had gripped my entire being and lifted me to a place far above any negative influence. It was joy unspeakable! The little children were dancing and praising God out of their pure and innocent hearts. This touched my heart. God is love. If you really seek Him from your heart, His love will be revealed to you, and you will never forget it. Forsake sin and receive the love of God today. "For God so loved the world that He gave His only begotten Son, that whosoever believes on Him should not perish but have everlasting life." #redeemingthetime

James 5:16; Psalm 22:3; 1 John 2:27; John3:16

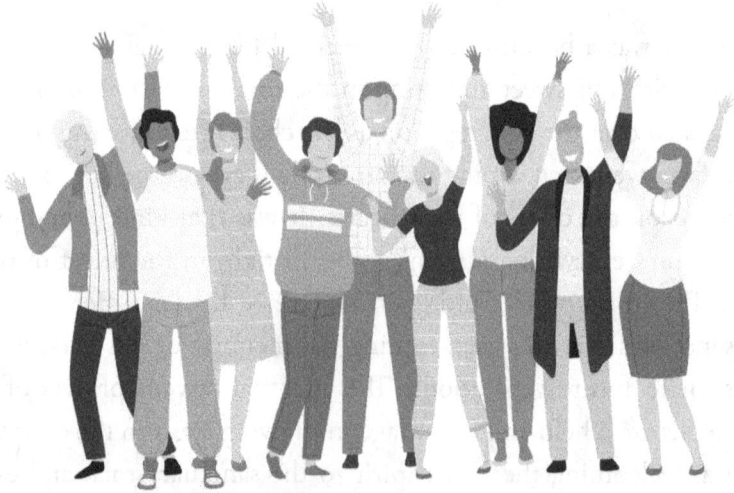

God Is Able

Let's see. You delivered me from being driven off a cliff. You spared my life when faced with a crazy dude with a gun. You didn't let me die when doctors had me smoking Asthmador cigarettes at the age of 12. You protected me in the Central storeroom showers guarding adult male prisoners. Because of you I have survived asthma, a heart murmur, atrial fibrillation, a T-6 lytic lesion on my spine and bone cancer.

All the glory belongs to you, dear God. Thank you for lifting my spirit today from a very low place and reminding me of your mercy and love. I can say like David, "For you have been a shelter for me and a strong tower from the enemy." "The salvation of the righteous is of the Lord." "He is their strength in the time of trouble." Trust God and His Word today. #redeemingthetime

Psalm 39:39; Psalm 61:3; Hebrews 4:16; Psalm 27:7

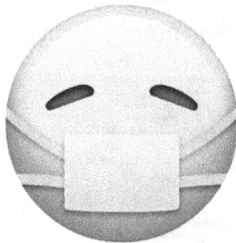

God Is Good

In this one of many "SNOW STORIES" I'm giving God the glory! A few days before the big event, a slight pain developed in my heart area. I shrugged it off as indigestion or a side effect of medication. Two days and 26 inches into the snow event I woke up in pain, with added pressure in my chest. At that point I called the paramedics, who in turn were assisted by the National Guard.

They arrived first on the scene as a team equipped with shovels to dig me out. The paramedic jumped through the snow in the process to assist me. By the time he was finished with his assessment the National Guard had dug a clear path to my home. They transported me to the Humvee and down the street to the waiting ambulance.

I am ever so grateful for the dedication and commitment that our local, statewide and federal agencies display in times of emergencies and extenuating circumstances. They need our prayers.

These young people got a lot of "thank you, baby" and "God bless you" while en route to the hospital, and an invitation to church. Thank you all for your continued prayers.

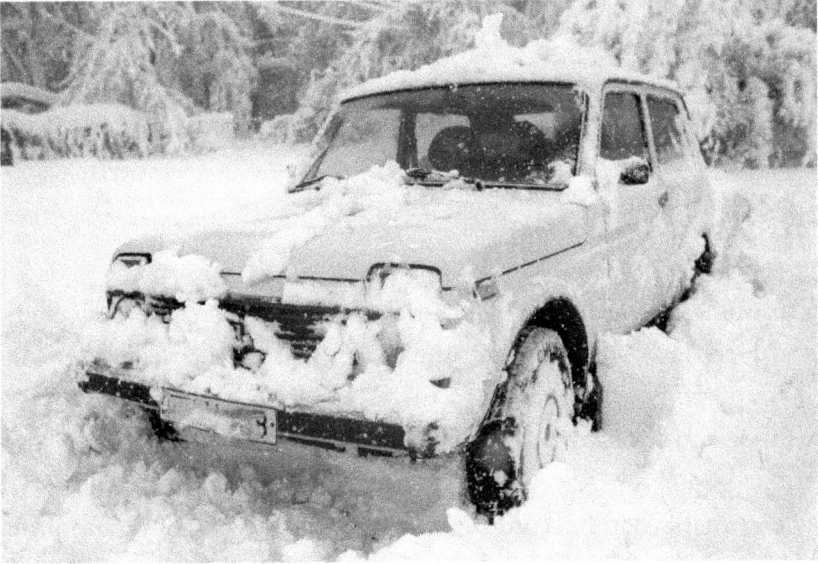

God Is Not Dead

Trusting God means knowing that God's plans are the best plans, and He knows what's around the corner and up the road. There are many reasons why things happen in our lives, but we have a God who can turn our dark days and deepest valleys into glorious outcomes. Sometimes we cry and ask "why." God knows all about your situation and according to his plans, the outcome will bring glory to Himself and knowledge to others that He exists and is real. #redeemingthetime

Romans 5:1-4; 1 Peter 4:12-14

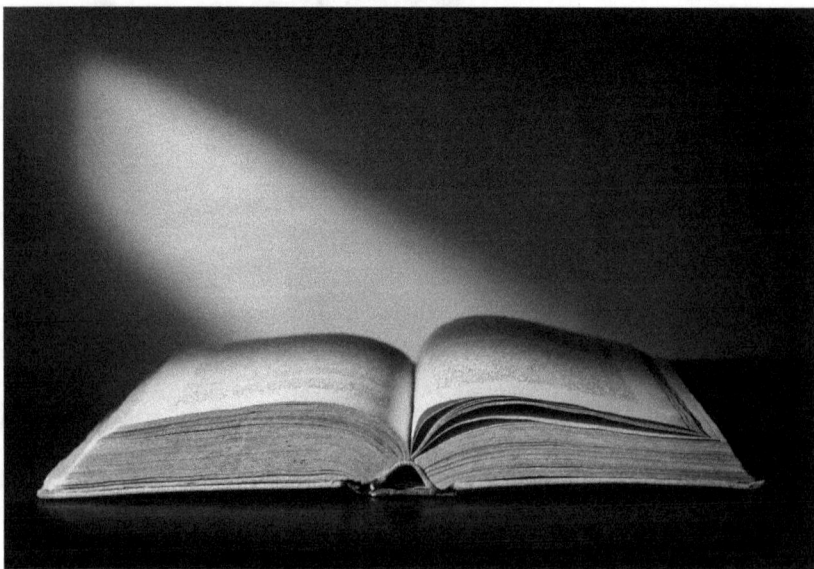

God Of The Universe

I am blown away by how BIG our God is. I have never seen Him. Ezekiel had a vision of Him being carried on His throne by heavenly creatures. Scientists have been able to look through the famous Hubble telescope and other powerful scopes to explore the Universe. Our home here on Earth is a speck compared to the size of our sun: 1.3 million Earths can fit inside of our huge sun. To top that, there is a humongous star out there that can house 6.8 million of our suns. This takes my breath away when I think of God and His wonderful works! The galaxy that we live in called the Milky Way includes our Sun, Moon, Planets and Stars. For years it was believed this was the extent of the universe. These huge telescopes reveal millions of other galaxies. Where am I going with this?

Scripture tells us that the Lord by wisdom founded the Earth; by understanding has He established the Heavens. What further blows me away in light of this scientific information is that God chose the speck of the Earth out of the humongous and numerous creations to establish His plan for mankind. In the beginning was the Word of God that became flesh and dwelt among us.

In our minute existence, God came in the flesh to redeem us back to Him. He hears us and sees us when we call upon Him. Receive and commit your life to God, the Maker of the Universe. For God so loved the world that He gave His only begotten Son (Jesus Christ) that whosoever believes in Him should not perish but have everlasting life. There is a plan for your life here on Earth as well as in God's heavenly kingdom. #redeemingthetime

Ezekiel Chapter 1; Proverbs 3:19; Genesis Chapter 1; St. John 1:1-14; 1st John 5:15; St. John 3:16; St. Luke 24:45-47; St. John 14:2D

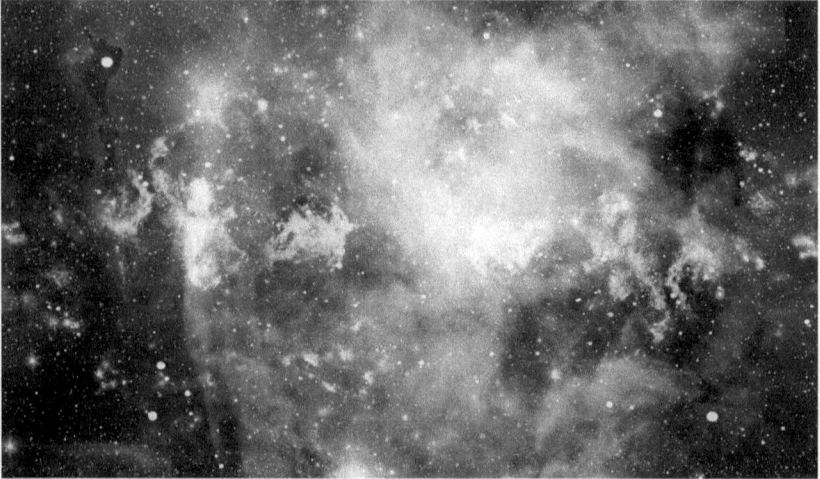

God's War

The battle is not yours; it's the Lord's. We hear this a lot, in messages and even in song. God himself stepped in on many wars and battles fought by his people, the Israelites. It is written that when they cried unto God in the battle, and put their trust in him, he heard their plea and came to the rescue. Their enemies were slain, sometimes on a massive scale, because the war was of God.

We as the people of God can still cry out to him and trust him when faced with adversity. Sometimes when we are flat on our backs with no hope in sight, we can look up and see God. Then we can cry unto him and trust him to fight our battles. When he answers by his immutable (never-changing Word), we rejoice in that we found out by experience that his Word is true. Our battles are not our own. It is God's war. Many are the afflictions of the righteous, but God delivers him out of them all. We can go from victory unto victory in every encountered battle. God gives us victory through our Lord Jesus Christ. Trust Him. #redeemingthetime

1 Chronicles 5:20-22; Psalm 34:19-22; 1 Corinthians 15:57; Romans 8:37

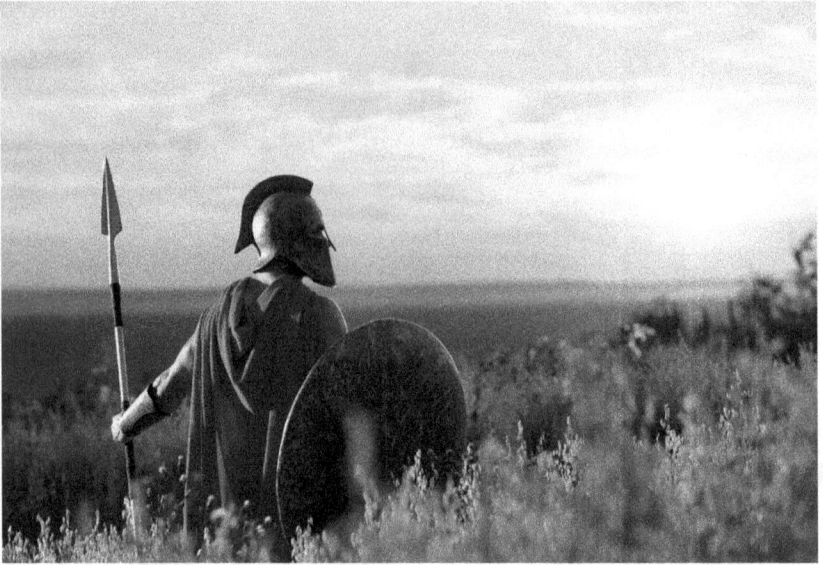

God's Got Something Good

I couldn't wait to get to the computer to share this encounter. While on vacation I caught a cold, which unfortunately turned into a full-blown asthma attack. With a weak immune system, I followed up at the hospital to receive antibiotics, steroids and other meds for relief. While there, I met 89-year-old Elizabeth, who had been dropped off a month ago for treatment and was never retrieved by guardians. A small, frail lady with a big heart and nothing but kind words just touched the heart of everyone who cared for her. I went over to introduce myself and was soon engaged in a conversation about her family.

My brother bought his computer to the hospital for use during my stay, which allowed me to assist Elizabeth. As a result, we were able to get a message out to her son. I was convinced that I was not going to leave the hospital until I shared the love of Jesus with her. As soon as I walked over, she extended her hand and gripped mine tightly, as if she knew my intentions. I said, "Elizabeth, do you know Jesus?" And she said, "He is a friend of mine. I was standing on the corner one day and out of the corner of my eye I saw a figure of a man coming my way. He kept coming straight to me. He told me, 'Jesus said your name is written on high. He told me to tell you your name will never be removed.' He is my friend and He is in my heart." I was moved to tears to know that God let Elizabeth know in spite of all her troubles she is not alone, and that God is mindful of all she is going through. We talked, laughed and praised God as she broke out in song: "This little light of mine; I'm gonna let it shine." Our room was full of joy and gladness, with some of the staff looking on. Please keep Ms. Elizabeth in your prayers. Behind every dark cloud, God's got something good for you.

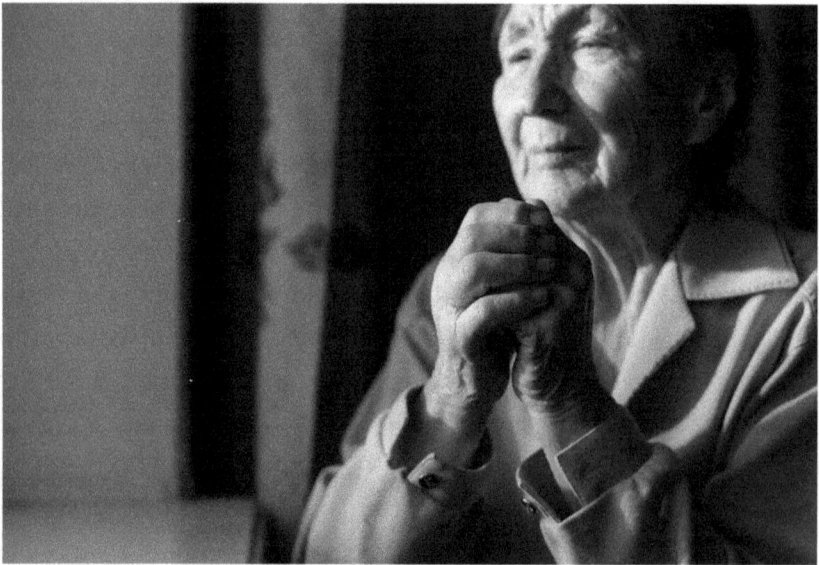

God's Sufficient Grace

No doubt there are some people, religions, and faiths that believe keeping the Ten Commandments justifies an entrance into Heaven. For years as a church member, I thought I was eligible and tried every day to be a good person. But I always found myself asking for forgiveness, doing wrong, making the wrong decisions and saying "I'm sorry" to others. I thought I was a Christian doing my best for God. It wasn't until I accepted God's love gift Jesus Christ into my life and repented of my sins that I was able to live according to God's will. The Christian walk has its challenges due to our ever-present adversary, Satan. He tries to discredit the plan of God for all and keep many from the truth of God's grace.

The Apostle Paul established numerous churches during his time, resulting in many conversions and an acceptance of Jesus Christ. They were nurtured in the ways of salvation and matured as new Christians. Paul was challenged to exhort the established church about receiving "another gospel." In his letter to the church, he was surprised that some were so soon removed from the truth of God's grace to another gospel. In those days, Jewish agitators had circulated among Gentile converts, seeking to impose circumcision and the burden of the Mosaic Law upon them as necessary for salvation.

As a new convert, I recall traveling home on the transit bus, singing and enjoying Jesus. A woman sitting across from me asked, "Where are your stockings?" Her suggestion was if I loved the Lord that much,

I should be covered. I don't recall my response, but I thank God He kept loving me and keeping me down through the years, minus the stockings. Today there are many things outside of Mosaic Law that are imposed upon Christians to challenge their faith in God. Paul intercepted and challenged the bondages that the Jewish Christians tried to impose. He exhorted, "Do I now persuade men or God? Or do I seek to please men? For if I yet pleased men, I should not be the servant of Christ." He told them they had been bewitched. They had stopped obeying the truth and were living in the flesh.

What has challenged your initial faith in God today, that you have returned to living in bondages and in the flesh? Are you believing man or God? Have you changed your mind about God's laws because of laws passed by government? Are you now living in the flesh because someone said it's ok, and everybody's doing it? As Paul exhorted the church, "Let us not be weary in well doing, for in due season we shall reap if we faint not."

Galatians 1:6-8; Gal. 1:10; Gal 3:1; Gal. 4:16; Gal. 4:9-10; Gal. 6:9,13

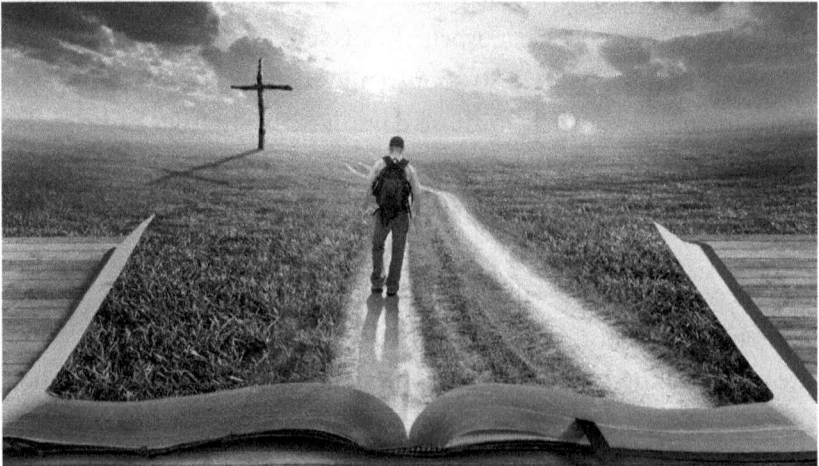

God's Grace

Don't let the Sanballats in your life distract you from your commission and heavenly goal. An interesting account in the Word of God speaks of a man by the name of Sanballat. He was one of the first to rise in rank among the people in Samaria, where there had been a long-running dispute among Samaritans and Jews. They disagreed over the location as to where God should be worshipped: in Mount Gerizim or in Jerusalem. When he heard that God's servant Nehemiah came to rebuild the walls of Jerusalem for the welfare of God's people, he became agitated and angry. He and his "gang" (as some historians view it) did all they could do to hinder and stop the work. A prophet was hired by Sanballat to lie against Nehemiah to bring a false report and criticism against him. He was ridiculed and mocked before the people and threatened with imminent attacks of war.

Nehemiah was a praying man, and one who fasted and sought counsel from God. In spite of the situation, he remained focused on the work and plan of God. Nehemiah was the king's cupbearer. His dedication to God and God's people caused him to obtain favor with the current king, who assisted him with his plan to go to Jerusalem to rebuild the walls. He encouraged the people to remain faithful to God, who would fight for and deliver them from the adversary. Sanballat failed in his attempts to stop the rebuilding of the walls of Jerusalem.

God's grace is sufficient for all that we encounter and experience on this Christian journey. Trust God that the situations and plots that come against you will fail. Know that the work God has called you to do will prosper and will bring forth what God designed it to do. God is not pleased with our holy wars, false accusations, and disputes against one another. Remain focused on the work you are called to do. The Sanballats we encounter are useful only for character building in the child of God. A good response to a bad situation builds character. #redeemingthetime

Nehemiah Chapters 1-4; 2 Corinthians 12:9; John 4:19-24

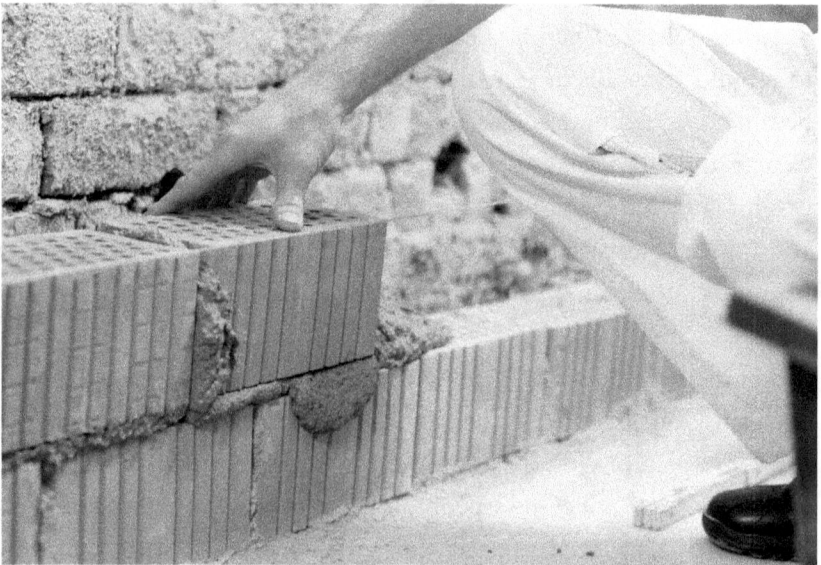

God's Mercy

I went in prayer today petitioning God for answers. Some days I have to give social media and current events a break just to recover from the overwhelming ongoing debacle that generates so much tragedy and rage. The struggle is real when putting my own two cents in on topics, particularly injustices, without becoming so intense as to enrage others.

I take comfort in knowing that everything going on in the world is in God's hands. Timothy, the Apostle of Jesus Christ, said it best: "This know also, that in the last days perilous times shall come. For men shall be lovers of their own selves, covetous, boasters, proud, blasphemers, disobedient to parents, unthankful, unholy, without natural affection, trucebreakers, false accusers, incontinent, fierce, despisers of those that are good, traitors, heady, high-minded, lovers of pleasures more than lovers of God; having a form of godliness but denying the power thereof" (2 Timothy 3: 1-5, KJV).

Reflecting back on my life, I realize I was once a part of the debacle until my life was changed by a merciful and forgiving God. The Lord our God is merciful and forgiving even though we have rebelled against him. He looked beyond my fault and saw my need. Though my sins were like scarlet, he made them as white as snow. Fall upon God's mercy and grace today. "For God so loved the world, that he gave his only begotten Son, that whosoever believes in him should not perish but have everlasting life." #redeemingthetime

John 3:16; Isaiah 1:18; 2 Corinthians 5:17; Daniel 9:9; Psalm 103:12; 2 Timothy 3:1-13

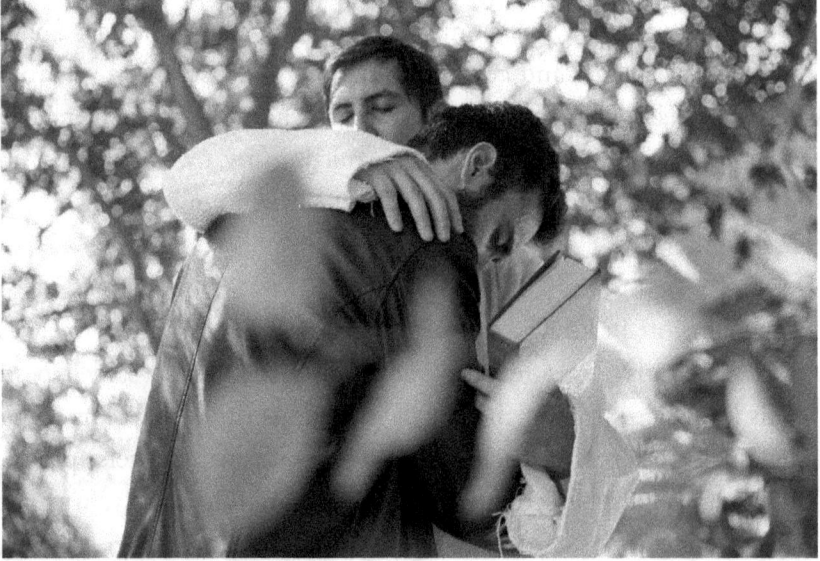

God's Mercy Extended

It's good to remember Lot's wife. If there ever is a time to remember, this is it. The sin of homosexuality had greatly polluted the cities of Sodom and Gomorrah before their destruction. Let us also remember the mercy of God. He left his heavenly abode to come and see if the sin was as bad as He was told. God was willing to spare the cities if there were any righteous ones left in it.

That tells me that God cares about the lost, even that very last one who would turn from their evil ways. His mercy endures forever. Let's remember that and be about the business of winning souls. #redeemingthetime

Psalm 100:5

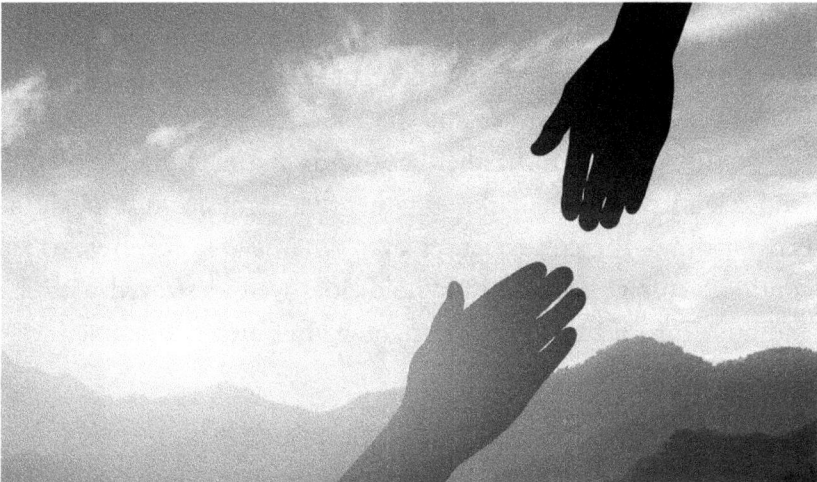

God's Plan

"Bone of my bone and flesh of my flesh" were the words expressed by the first man God created, named Adam. The Almighty God of the universe, the heavens and the earth formed man from the dust of the ground. It was a decision made by God with other Heavenly Hosts to create male and female after their image and likeness to be fruitful, multiply and replenish the earth.

Adam's companion Eve, the first female, was created from the rib of Adam. God opened Adam's flesh after putting him in a deep sleep and took out one of his ribs. After closing the flesh, He created Eve, calling her woman because she was created from man. Adam and Eve were husband and wife, designed by God's magnificent plan to populate the earth. As it was then, it is so now that a man leaves his father and mother and cleaves to his wife so that they shall be one flesh.

Now that we have knowledge of our existence and purpose, the Almighty Creator has left the door open by giving us a right to choose His way, our way or the way of destruction. As we can see, the world has gone all together backwards and far from the plan of God. Men have chosen darkness rather than light down through the eons of time. The consequences over time have been severe as sin continues to rage among us. Whole cities were destroyed with fire and brimstone because men were going after men and women were going after women for sex.

If you have fallen into this trap and been tricked by our adversary Satan, there is hope and mercy for you. You don't have to be a part of the judgment and consequences for sin. God's mercy has endured even though he's angry with the wicked every day.

"For God so loved the world that he gave his only begotten Son, that whosoever believes in him should not perish but have everlasting life." Trust God to give you a new life. Repent. Give Jesus Christ your heart today by repeating this simple prayer: Lord Jesus, forgive me of all of my sins. Wash me clean in the blood that you shed for me on the cross of Calvary. Come into my heart today. I receive you as my Savior and I confess you as my Lord. To know and learn more about your decision for Christ, you are invited to attend Faith Tabernacle Church 2422 West Patapsco Ave. Baltimore, MD 21230 Join us on Sundays at 11:00 am for morning worship. #redeemingthetime

Psalm 103:14; Psalm 100:3; Genesis 1:26-28; Genesis 2:21-25; John 3:16; Psalm 7:11; Genesis 19:1-29

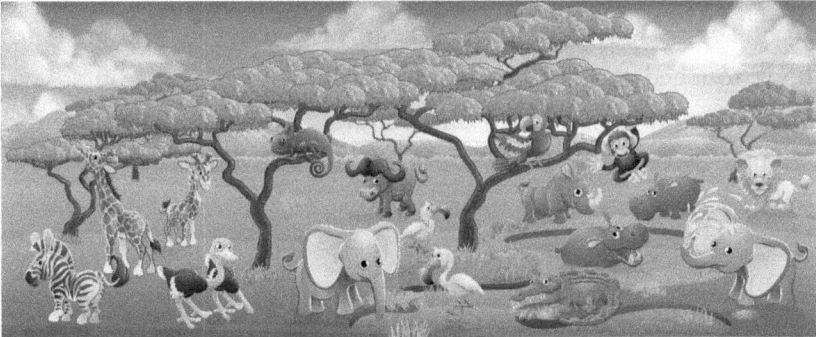

God Is Still In Control

There is so much to pray about, cry about, and travail about as the entire world seems to be turned upside down. Today my prayer began with tears for the 68 prisoners burned up in a jail station house in Venezuela. I thought of my own son, who is also incarcerated, and how I would feel if this tragedy had happened here. Facebook and other social media provide a world of information and sharing at every level of life. It reveals the hearts and minds of everyone who shares a thought or message. Some posts are painful to read but provide me with more reason to stay in the prayer closet. As of today, 250 million people are using Facebook. It is a mass world of harvest for those of us who see the opportunities to defend our faith, share the love of God and be a witness for Christ.

As the windows of Heaven were opened today in prayer, God's heart touched mine while petitioning Him to open the blind eyes and hearts of men women and children everywhere. God's mercy endures forever, and He is concerned for the lost. I get angry and sometimes enraged over the things that our adversary does via the vessels he controls here on earth. Then I have to realize that those vessels are blind to that fact that they are under his control. Nothing is too hard for God. Share the Gospel. God is concerned for the lost. #redeemingthetime

2 Corinthians 4:4; John 12:38-40; 2 Peter 3: 8-10; Psalm 100:5

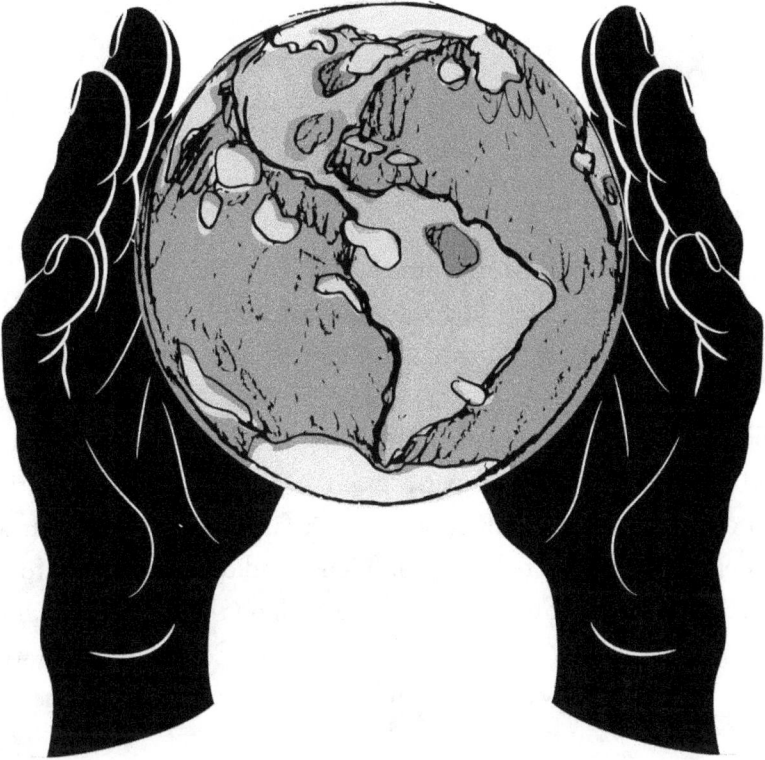

God's Way

"It is a fearful thing to fall into the hands of the living God." This is a scripture from the Bible admonishing and instructing the early church on how to avoid the judgments of God. The author spoke of many who despised the Law of Moses and died without mercy under two or three witnesses. The New Testament church members and converts experienced persecution in the form of humiliation, reproaches, terror and affliction for their faith in Jesus Christ. It was evident that some were losing confidence and drawing back into sin. The author spoke of those who turned back on the Lord and counted his sacrifice on the cross as an unholy thing. Considering the work of God as unholy was worthy of worse punishment, as in the days of Moses.

God smote Miriam with leprosy, comparing her murmuring against Moses to a father spitting on the face of his daughter. In those days, it was a custom to spit on a person's face as a gesture of disgust and shame. Therefore, God set Miriam out of the camp seven days to be ashamed for seven days. His mercy brought her back into the camp after a week's time. This is one of the more merciful accounts of God's mercy. The author is admonishing the early church members and converts not to cross the line when turning back and speaking against the work of God. God is the same yesterday, today and forever. His mercy also endures forever.

Still, there are those in the church, as in the days of old, "plucking God's nerves" with conversations and plots against his anointed servants and his work. Moses pleaded with God to be merciful to Miriam, but she had gone too far. God has no pleasure in those who turn back to sin and purposely discredit his Work. The just and righteous of God live by Faith. Don't be one of those who turn back, but be one of those who believe to the saving of the soul. #redeemingthetime

Numbers 12:1-15; Hebrews 10:26-39

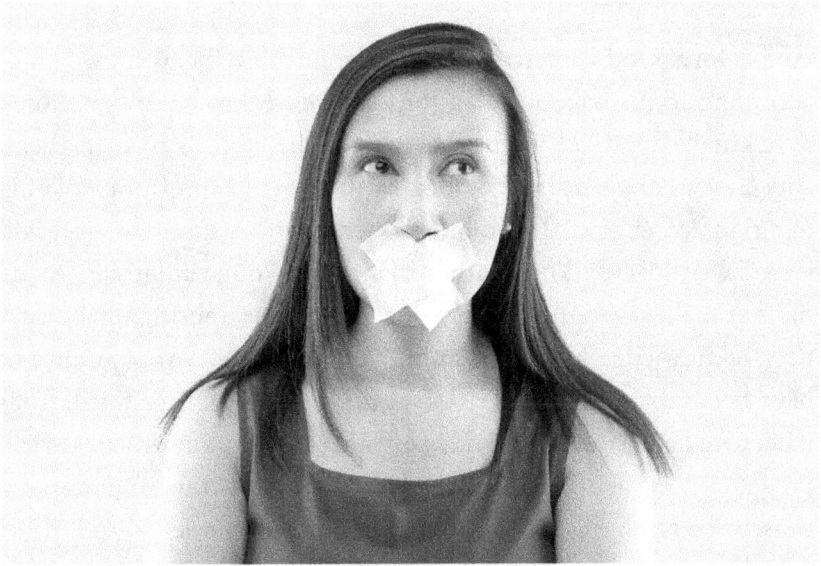

God Understands

"Help me to understand why God would allow me to suffer so much abuse as a child by a parent who was supposed to love and nurture me." Response:

God is love. God is merciful. God responds to the choices we make according to his will and plan for our lives. Many have not chosen to acknowledge God in their lives or invite him in to help them. Any choices made outside of God's will prevent Him from violating our right of choice. The Bible says choose this day who you will serve. Men love darkness rather than light. Your parent apparently did not make the right choices concerning your upbringing, nor did they acknowledge God concerning you. Otherwise, you would not have been abused. I am so sorry for the abuse you suffered. Your parent made decisions that not only affected you but others as well. However, God acts in his Divine Providence, touching the hearts of those who reach out to the abused, neglected, homeless and more. It is the daily prayers of the Saints of God that petition him to send relief, provision and protection in matters such as these. And unfortunately, there are many who don't have anyone to call their name out in prayer.

You have God to thank for your life and that you are still here. Your life is a testimony that may help someone in their situation. Renew your commitment to God. Confess every sin and receive Jesus as your personal Savior and Lord. There are exceeding great and precious promises to the child of God who is operating inside the will of God. He loves you and wants to use you. Then you will be able to forgive. Forgiveness will free your mind and lift you higher in God's will (Matthew 6:14-15).

Father, touch us today with your love. Give us a heart of forgiveness and a hunger and thirst for righteousness in the name of Jesus. #redeemingthetime

PEOPLE NEED THE LORD. BE A WITNESS AND AMBASSADOR FOR CHRIST.

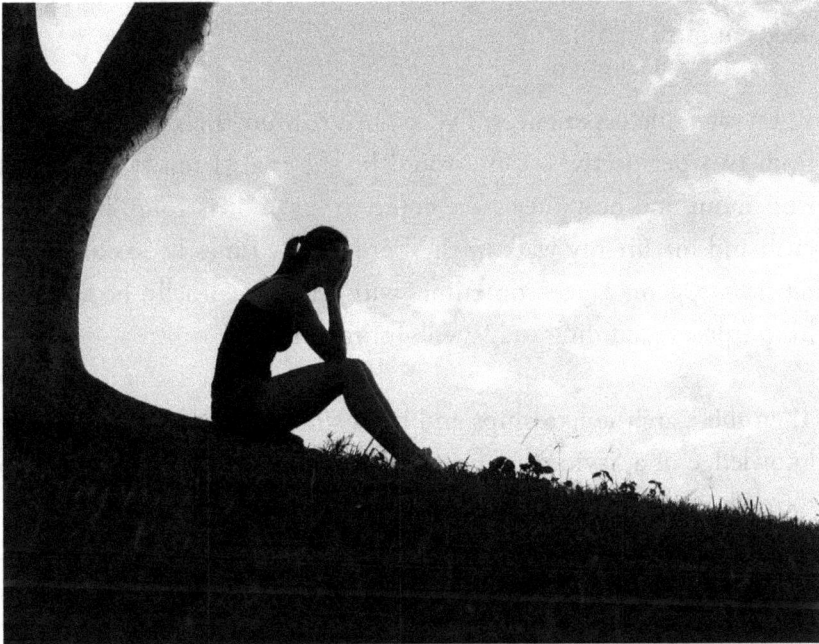

People Need The Lord

"Dear God, what's happening to me?"... is the statement made by the younger version of Whoopi Goldberg's portrayal in the movie *Color Purple*. She is the pre-teen with two children by her stepfather, (given away) and seen walking behind her mother's casket, asking God questions. However entertaining, the movie captures the reality of post slavery hardships and family life in the early 20's and 30's. There was much suffering to endure in those days and a lack of basic needs in most families.

In my own life experiences, I've learned to view trials and hardships from two perspectives. One would be the trials I testify, read, and sing about and how they have come to make me strong, boost my faith and mature my walk in the Lord. Many times I've asked God, *what's happening to me?* sometimes with tears. Eventually, he revealed his purpose, according to his will, for my life.

Then there are the hardships and trials suffered by those lacking the knowledge of a Savior in Christ Jesus with nowhere to turn or who to reach out to for help. In most cases they've been rejected by family, peers, and community. There are many creative ways within and without the church to reach the lost in this age of God's grace. We as Christians have the answer to, "Dear God, what's happening to me?"

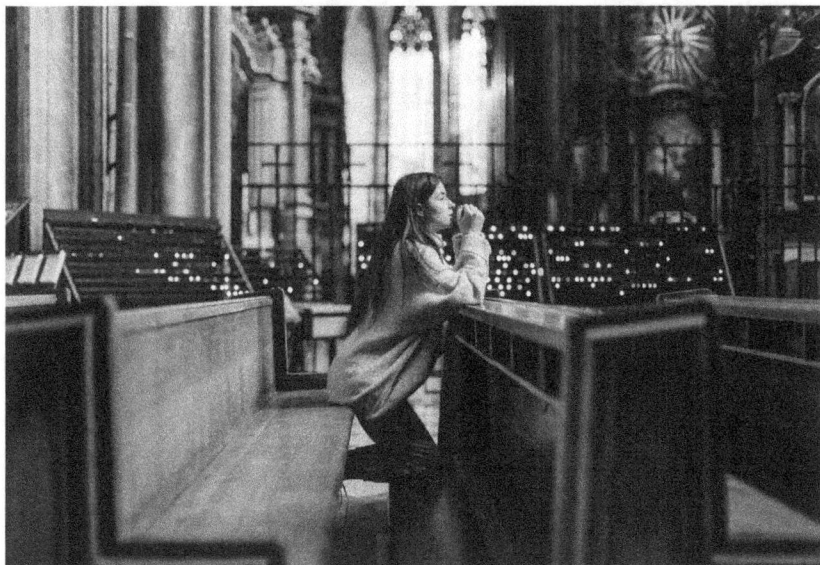

Good News

He (Jesus) was BRUISED for OUR INIQUITIES (sins). It was unimaginable pain. For what? Why? Because He LOVES us and doesn't want us to end up in an eternal lake of fire. Which sin is more brazen than the other? He was bruised for all of them. LIFT JESUS UP! He said, "If I be lifted up, I will draw all men unto me."

When you come out of your prayer closet with the anointing, arm yourself with the Good News that Jesus saves. It's the anointing that breaks the yoke. Ultimately, going to the polls can change a lot of things, but prayer and its answer are the keys.

Fret not yourself because of evildoers. Keep praying for them because we were evildoers once. Let God be God. His MERCY still endures forever. He is our JUDGE.

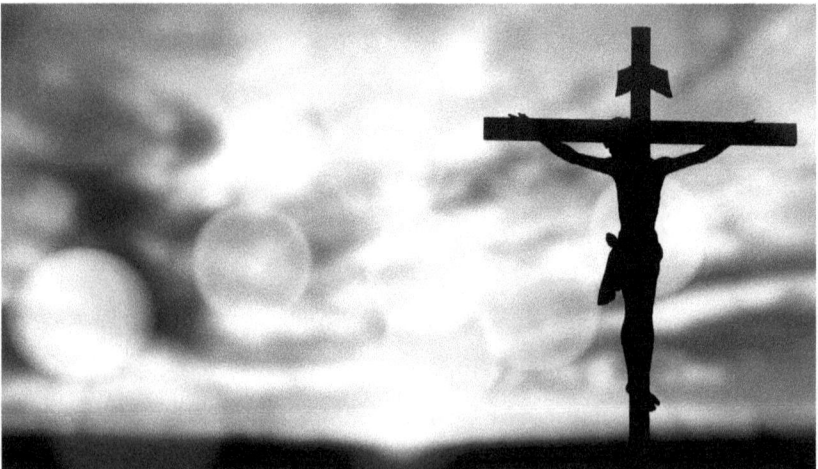

Habitat Of Doves

One day in my Christian experience, I was discouraged and ready to call it quits. For a whole month I wrestled with anger, hurt and disappointment. I had decided I was going to keep it to myself because I didn't want anyone to become a victim of my discontent.

I eventually confided in someone who I knew would take the matter into prayer. We were on the porch on a warm, sunny day discussing the matter. Out of the blue a dove appeared on the awning of the neighbor's porch, staring right at us. It was beautiful, pure white in color with bright red eyes. My friend and I looked at each other and decided at that moment that I needed to put the matter in God's hands and not complain. The dove flew away not long after that statement was made.

The Bible tells Christians to be wise as serpents but harmless as doves in the world we live in. Our response to a matter should take into consideration how others may be affected. And God has a way of dealing with the offended as well as the offender to keep us on the same page and goal to make Heaven. I later learned that a dove's habitat is usually in open country and grasslands of the Central Prairie states. GOD WAS MINDFUL OF MY SITUATION AND SENT A DOVE all the way to Baltimore County, Maryland to deliver an illustrated message. #redeemingthetime

Matthew 10:16; James 1:19; Proverbs 15:1; Ephesians 4:26

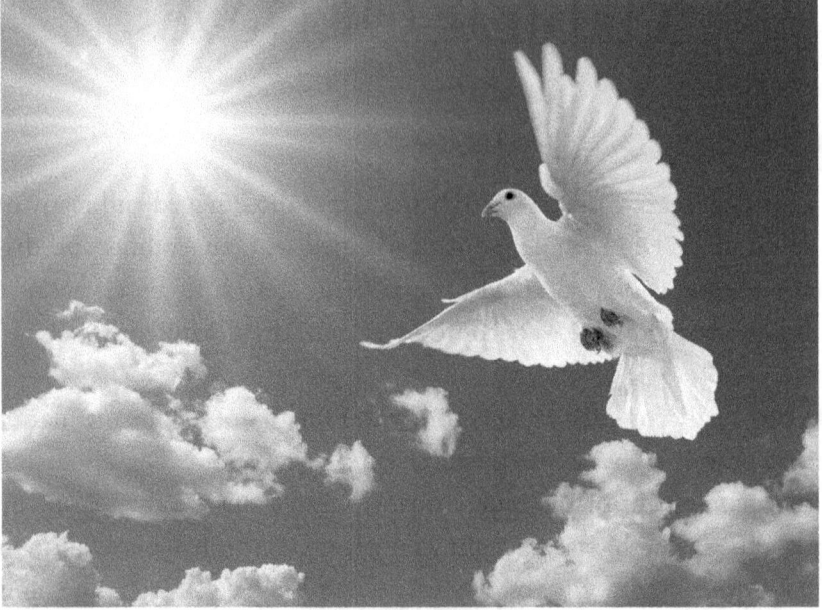

He Was There All The Time

Witnessing the moving of God's Holy Spirit is a sweet and heartfelt experience. The topic of this morning's Bible study was God's grace. Those present each shared an experience of God's grace in their lives and a testimony of his loving touch. One inspiring story brought tears to my eyes.

My friend and neighbor remembered going to a camp meeting at the age of seven. She found herself being led to the altar call. She wasn't sure what was happening to her but felt the power of God overcome her entire being. She had never felt anything like that. With tears in her eyes, she said to all of us, "I want it back!" With the lesson momentarily paused, God's sweet presence touched my friend and others who were listening.

Being touched by the spirit of the Almighty God is an unforgettable experience at any age. When God knocks on your heart's door, don't ignore it. God is calling you. #redeemingthetime

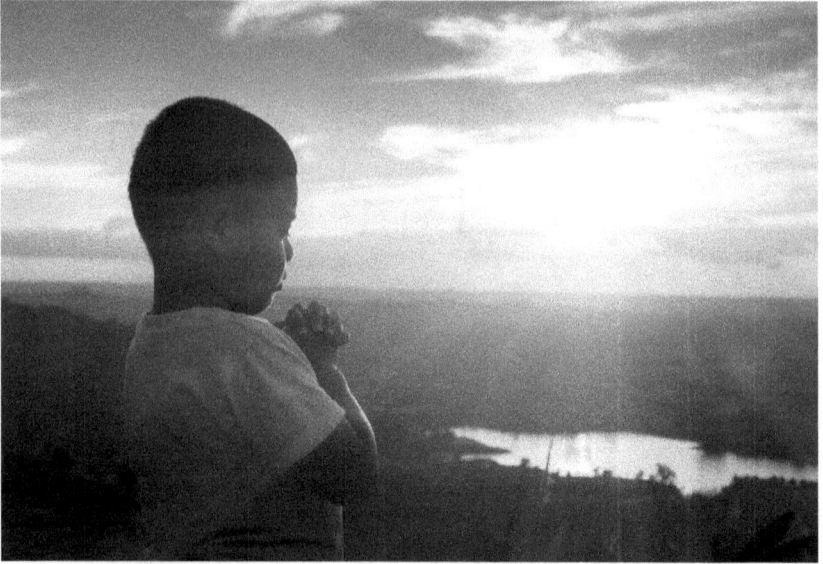

He Will Sustain You

Elijah obeyed God, who provided a brook for water and a raven to bring food during the drought. When the brook dried up Elijah further obeyed God and journeyed to a place where a widow was prepared to sustain him during the drought. The footsteps of the righteous are ordered by the Lord. Obey the voice of the Lord, and someone will be there to sustain you in your time of need.

1 Kings 17: 1-16

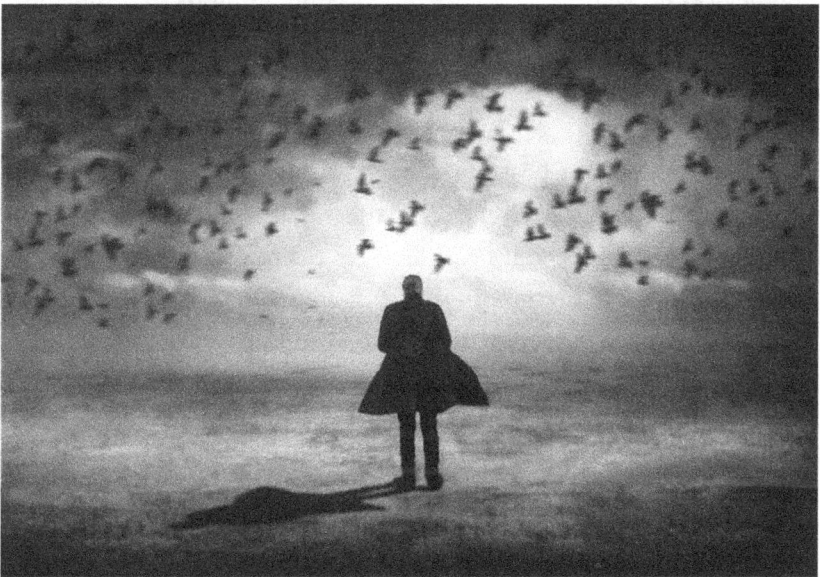

Hold Your Peace

It becomes increasingly hard to stay positive in the midst of so much bad and controversial news. Our minds as well as our health can become affected due to the details and nature of the same. There are also those issues and current events that we are passionate about, that carry varying opinions opposite of our own. Our adversary seeks avenues in the midst of it all to cause separation and division among us. How do I know? Many times, I struggle to hold my peace over issues relevant to my position, where I feel the opposing side is just flat out wrong. It is important to be vigilant about the manipulations and devices of Satan. He can use our varying opinions to bring about misunderstandings, controversies, and negative exchanges. He will cause us to look at one another differently because of our viewpoints.

Deciding to hold our peace is divinely inspired in order to keep the peace. It drives one to prayer over matters that would ordinarily cause us to act out of character. It helps us to see the needs of others who may fall victim to misunderstandings and discord. We become an integral part of building up the body of Christ as opposed to tearing it down. And, most important, the plan of Satan is thwarted. #redeemingthetime

Ephesians 4:3-13

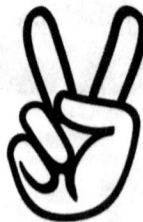

Holy Ghost And Fire

Long ago, I didn't know nothing about Jesus and His love. I used to sing this song whenever I visited my mother's church, followed by my testimony. The rest of the song is expressed by one of the marvelous moments experienced in God's presence tonight at my church.

The presence of the Lord approached in the midst of the praise service and throughout the exhortation and offering. As the tears started flowing, I knew the Lord was very near and taking me to a place far above worries and cares. As the minister called for a renewing and preparation for the ongoing work of the Lord, the prayers of the saints for one another released a connection that could barely be contained. My soul was on fire, the tears were flowing, and my body is still feeling the effects of the glory from Heaven that consumed the service tonight. I couldn't wait to get home to share this marvelous moment in the Lord with you. Get to know the Lord. He's good all the time!

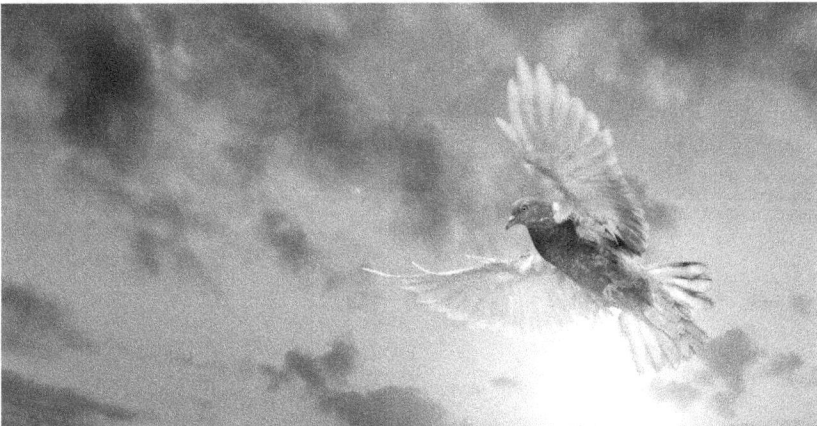

Intervene, Lord!

"THE VOICE OF THY BROTHER'S BLOOD CRIETH UNTO ME FROM THE GROUND." God was speaking to Cain when he was asked what he had done to his brother. In his anger, Cain killed his brother for cheating him out of his birthright.

There are a host of reasons why people are being killed today, including deception, theft, drugs, envy, money, etc., just to name a few. But my people, my brothers and sisters, are being killed because of the color of our skin. My people are also God's people. God asked Cain, "Where is thy brother?" Cain answered, "I know not, am I my brother's keeper?"

Someone knows how three black bodies ended up hanging from three trees within days of one another in America. God sees, God hears and God knows. My prayer is that these murders committed in secret be rooted out, holding those responsible accountable for their evil deeds.

"Keep us out of harm's way, oh God, and from seen and unseen dangers." Our blood being shed on the streets of America speaks to God. He will intervene. He will avenge. #redeemingthetime

Genesis: Chapter 4

I Saw The Light

Saul, the persecutor and murderer of Christians, and one who stood by and consented to Stephen's death, was stopped on the Damascus Road by a light brighter than the sun. A voice spoke out of that light and asked, "Why do you persecute me?" It was the voice of Jesus reasoning with Saul (who was later known as Paul) to ponder his own reasons for killing so many Christians during a great persecution of the church. This was a one-on-one important encounter where Paul's companions could only hear but not see Jesus. It resulted in Paul's salvation, conversion to Christianity and calling to the work of God. He was a chosen vessel to bear the name of Jesus to Jews, non-Jews and kings.

Paul, a government official who made havoc of the church, hauling men and women into prison for their faith in Jesus, stopped to consider the matter of his soul. He said, "What will you have me to do?" In his conversion process he was filled with the Holy Spirit and baptized. When I view world leaders and government officials of this day and time, I see them as potential Christians, who God can reason with to turn them around from their evil ways, as he did with Saul. The Apostle Paul was careful not to offend God or men while fulfilling his commission. He received favor on several occasions and was received by governors as a result. King Agrippa, the great grandson of Herod the Great, said, "Almost you persuade me to be a Christian." There are many ways to speak to our government officials as constituents and concerned Christians. Only God knows if an audience,

letter, or email of reasoning and persuasion will touch the heart of
_____ (You fill in the blank). #Redeemingthetime

Acts 8:1,3; Acts 9:1-18; Acts 24:16; Acts 25:7; Acts 26:12-18;
Matthew 2:1-23

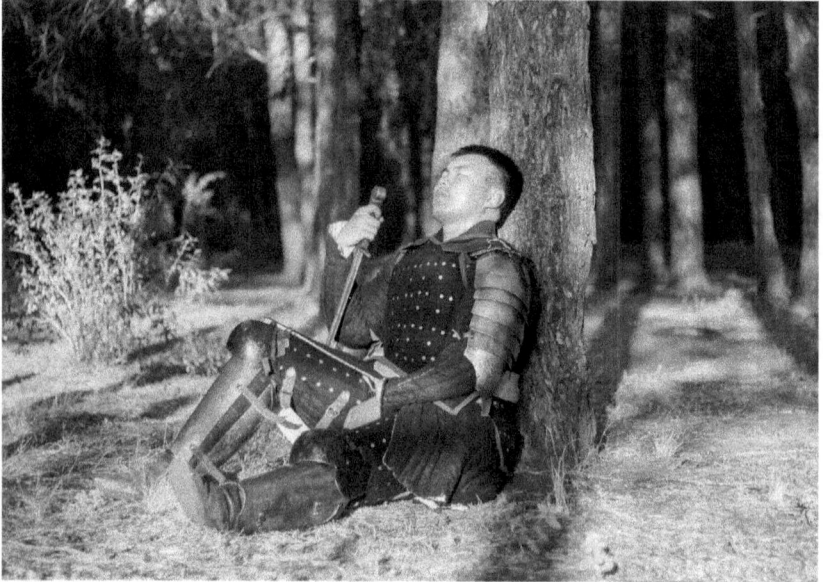

Jesus The Equalizer

Years ago, I was surprised to discover that some cemeteries appear to separate the indigent in burial. A relative who was very poor passed away in a hospice facility without insurance. The funeral home offered a low-cost package along with assistance in burial from the care facility. The burial took place in a beautiful location locally. However, when we arrived, we were directed to a remote area of the grounds far from and out of range from the grave sites and tombstones. I remember thinking, "are they expanding the cemetery or is this where they bury all the poor people?"

Although the latter thought seemed appropriate to the surroundings, things aren't always as they seem. Death becomes the equalizer to any and all attempts to separate or categorize in this life. In preparing for the next life the Almighty God requires your soul. Did you know that your body is like a tent surrounding your soul and spirit that will live on forever? Did you know there is a Heaven prepared for you, and a Hell not directly prepared for you? Hell was prepared for Satan and his angels, and Satan wants to take you there. The time is short. Evil is so prevalent in the earth.

You can escape the forces of evil against you and its consequences by turning to God. Get rid of the evil eyes against your brothers and sisters. Forgive often. Drop the titles and name calling. Stop the lying, the cheating, the hate and giving God the finger. He sees all that you do. Yet he is compassionate, his mercy endures forever, and he loves you. "For God so loved the world that he gave his only begotten Son, that whosoever believeth in him should not perish, but have everlasting life." (John 3:16, KJV)

Take charge of your future destination and get right with God today. Pray this simple prayer. *Lord. Be merciful to me, a sinner. Wash me in your blood that you shed on Calvary's Cross for me. Forgive me of all of my sins. I receive you as my Savior and confess you as my Lord.* Connect and reconnect with God at your local household of faith. If you don't have a church home you are welcome at Faith Tabernacle Church, 2422 West Patapsco Avenue, Baltimore, MD, 21230 Meet with us Sundays, for 11am Worship Service and more.

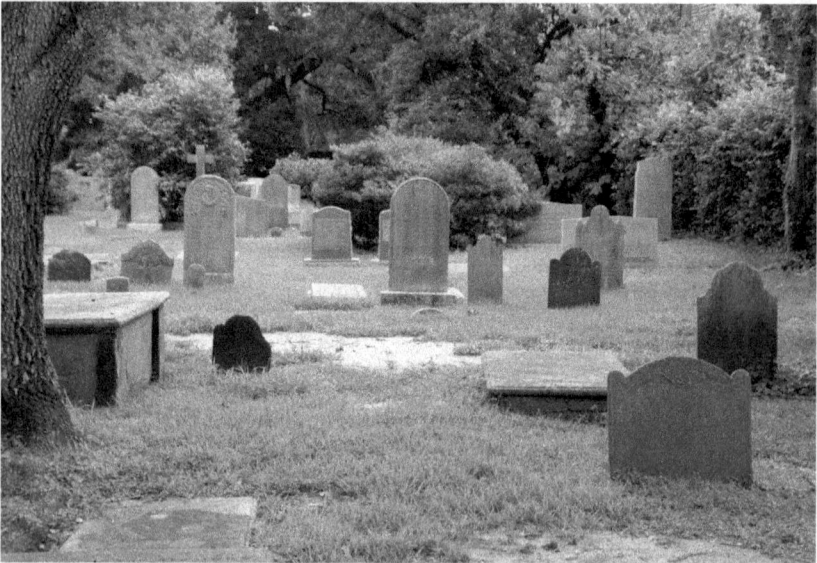

Jesus Is Love

I was 21 and in love, and thought I was being loved until I became pregnant. Things were going ok until it was suggested by my boyfriend at the time that I "get rid of it." Although I don't remember all the details of the conversation, the whole scenario eventually led me to the abortion doctor with my boyfriend present. Love led me all the way to the doctor's office, but my conscience wouldn't let me go through with it. Before I could express my feelings, the doctor advised us he was no longer performing abortions. I was so relieved, but my boyfriend called it quits after I told him I did not want to try another doctor. Come to find out, there was someone else in the picture.

In those days "get rid of it" meant finding someone to perform an abortion illegally. Someone was praying for me. Looking back, I realize my mind was blinded by foolish love and bad decisions. I made two choices that day: first to go to the doctor, and second, to decide against the abortion. I didn't know God then, but God knew me. I'm paying it forward. My prayer today is for all who are struggling with decisions for many reasons concerning abortion. Maybe you had one or more for whatever reason and can't seem to forgive yourself. You are loved by the Almighty Creator. He will not condemn you. He loves you. "For God so loved the world, that he gave his only begotten Son Jesus Christ, that whosoever believes on him should not perish but have everlasting life." God loves you and will forgive you. Father, touch hearts today with your love. Let them know that you forgive, just with the asking. Lead and guide them to a place of refuge in the name of Jesus. #redeemingthetime

John 3:16-17

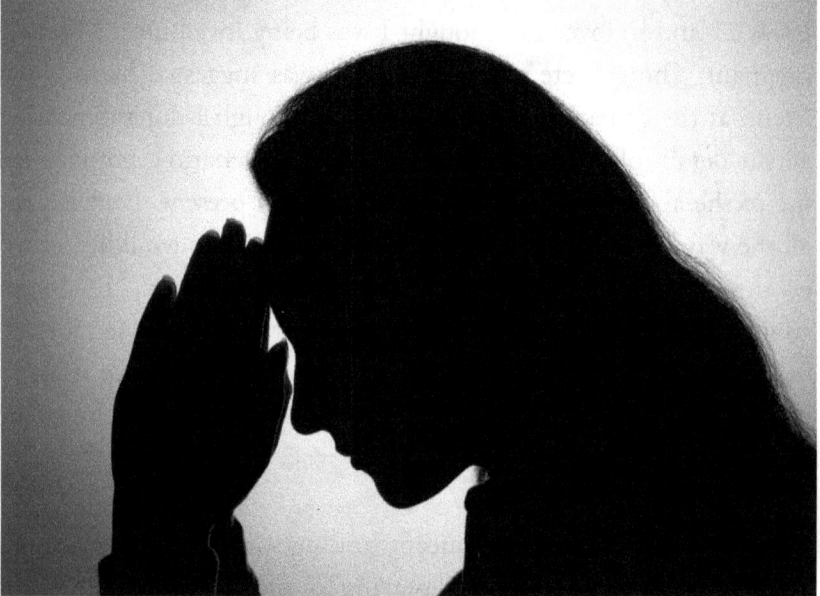

Answer The Call

Heaven came down and glory filled my soul one night in 1972. I went to a meeting one night and my heart wasn't right. Something got a hold on me. That something wasn't a thing at all. It was the glorious love of God filling my soul after I repented of my sins. A faithful friend invited me to church after convincing me of my need for salvation. At the time, I thought I was ok with sinning a little bit and making up for it in church attendance every Sunday.

Little did I know that I was only doing what came naturally and that God was calling me back to him. It is written that by one man's sin we were all made sinners, but by one man's death on the cross of Calvary, we were all given the hope of eternal life. I was born to love God and receive his love gift to the world Jesus Christ. Not only did I receive him that night in 1972, but he also wrote my name in the Lamb's book of life. There is no need to wonder what your future holds. Receive Jesus Christ into your heart today. #redeemingthetime

John 3:16; Acts 4:12; Romans 5:12; Revelation 21:1-27

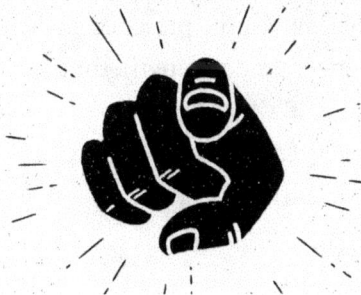

Judgment

So the whole Tribe of Benjamin was accused of lewdness and folly in Israel and refused to give up those among them who were responsible. Prior to abusing a woman all night long, ending in her death, they also attempted sodomy with a Levite, one who held various religious duties among the Israelites. This barbaric behavior caused God to extract them from the Tribes of Israel. Because they were left-handed men of valor with great marksmanship, they prevailed three times in battle against their brothers (the Israelites). As the Israelites continued to cry out to God, the Lord defeated Benjamin before Israel, twenty-five thousand and one hundred of them, leaving a remnant hiding in the wilderness. My heart is heavy over the many men, women and children, particularly Christians, dying horrible deaths in foreign lands at the hands of barbarian terrorists.

James said it well: "From whence come wars and fighting among you? Come they not hence even of your lusts that war in your members?" As we continue to cry out and pray against these atrocities, know that God is in control and will extract the unrepentant evildoers. All the skill, talent, success and status purported of the unregenerate— nothing will overshadow God's presence in bringing judgment on continued disobedience. #redeemingthetime

Judges Chapters 19, 20 & 21; James 4:1

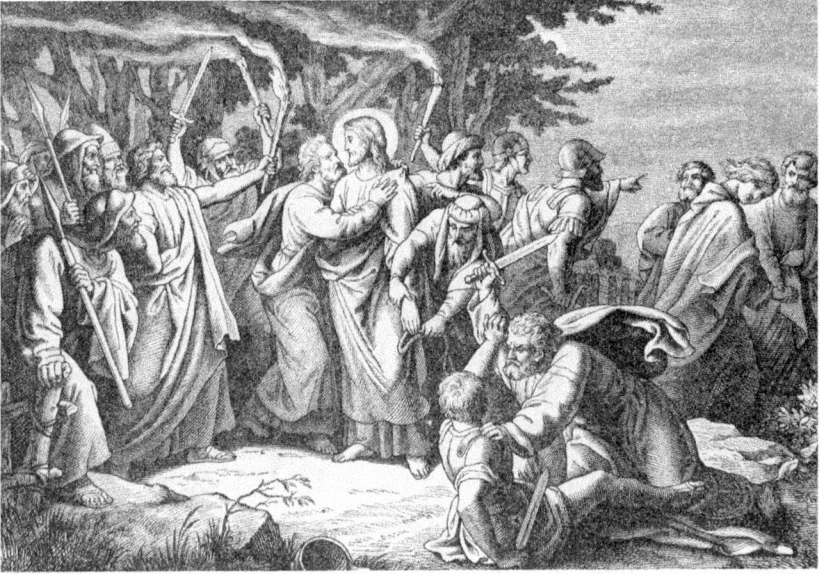

Keep Jesus First

I went to a County Wide Forensic Festival competing against other High Schools in Debate and Poetry Reading. I did a reading by Black poet Paul Lawrence Dunbar called ANTEBELLUM SERMON. This was spoken and written in dialect representative of slaves who couldn't read and were forbidden to read. My principal at the time was highly upset that my English teacher entered me into this competition. She did not want me to represent our school speaking in slave language. Coming back with a first-place win signified that many at that competition appreciated and understood the representation of and the effects of slavery.

To all graduates, BE THE BEST YOU CAN BE. DON'T LET ANYONE TELL YOU TO TAKE A BACK SEAT. If you're going off to college, keep Jesus first. Challenge those professors when they speak against God and promote evil. I did. You will be blessed!

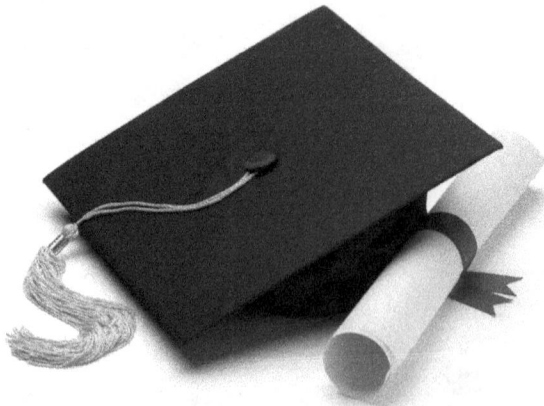

Keep Your Ship Afloat

The shipwreck of the *Costa Concordia* was a terrible tragedy. It was carrying over 4000 people when it deviated from its planned route and struck a rock formation on the sea floor. The tragedy created multiple ramifications, including the arrest of the captain for failure to assist passengers and abandoning the ship. It took over a month to recover and identify all of the deceased passengers. The ship was dismantled and materials from the ship were recycled. Paul encouraged Timothy to hold on to his faith and to pattern his life after the Lord Jesus Christ. He also made mention of those who made shipwrecks concerning their faith.

Our tests and trials as Christians are designed to mature us to completely place our trust in God and his Word. According to Paul, a shipwreck of our faith can be a tough learning experience. Going ahead of God and making our own decisions can cause failure. And those looking on us are affected. Consider that the things we say and do could turn people away from God. We are epistles known and read of all men. Keep your ship afloat. #redeemingthetime.

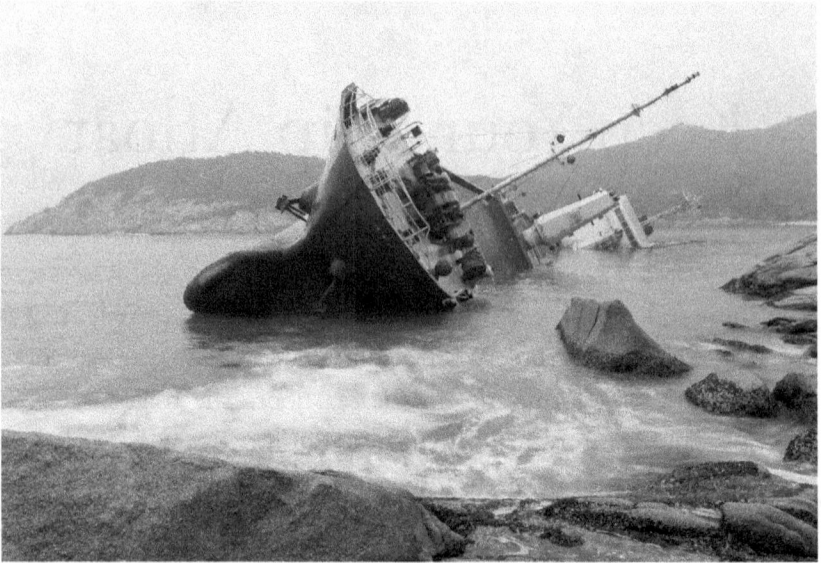

Know God, Know Peace

The sinking of the RMS Titanic is an event in history that has been depicted numerous times via Broadway, Cinema Screens, and other media. The historical account describes a Catholic Priest, Thomas Boyles, from England, as one of the passengers on the Titanic. He was portrayed consoling passengers during the ship's final moments. Also, the ship's Band Master and Violinist, Wallace Hartley, consoled the passengers with music as the ship began to sink. He led the Band with the final song *Nearer My God To Thee*.

In the fictional depiction of these historical characters, human nature's reaction, when faced with imminent doom, was real. The Priest was at peace with God and was able to console others. However, there were many who were looking for a blessing and a prayer from a man, crying and clutching his clothing and feet as if he could carry them to Heaven. The violinist was also at peace and played standing alone until the very end while the band members ran for their lives.

The Peace of God is Powerful and a wonderful Gift from Heaven. It doesn't appear overnight but comes through the many trials of life and the tight spots that God will bring you to and through. I read a sign once that said, NO GOD, NO PEACE. KNOW GOD, KNOW PEACE. It is a process. You need God to have this Peace. No doubt, Thomas Boyles and Wallace Hartley knew God. For God so loved the world that he gave his only begotten Son that whosoever believes on him should not perish but have everlasting life. Give Jesus your heart today and KNOW PEACE. #redeemingthetime

John14:27, Jeremiah 17:5, Philippians 4:7, John 3:16, Romans 10:9

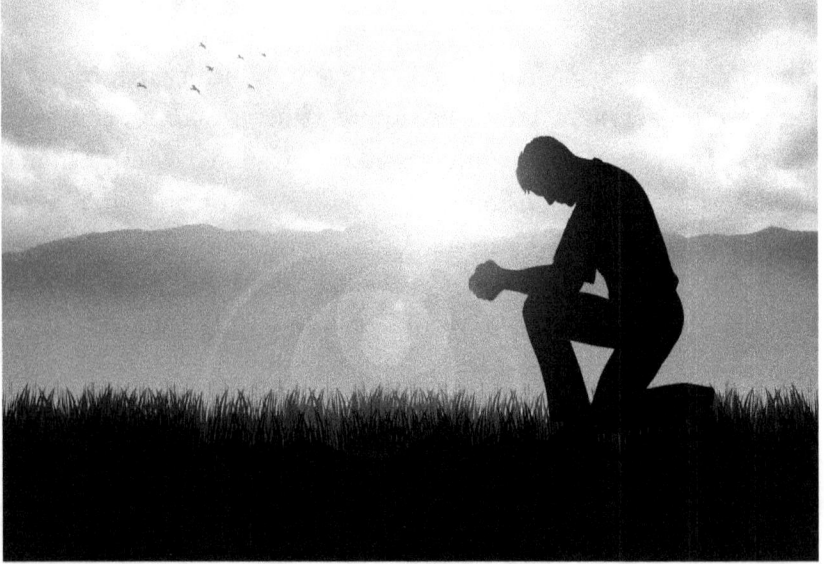

Lesson From God

My prayers are going up for the new President Elect Donald Trump. It will be interesting to see how God's agenda will be manifested via his tenure in office. Speaking on post-election results today comes with the responsibility of choosing words appropriate for divided and differing mindsets. Our response to any matter affects the hearer and what is spoken can be inspiring, insensitive, or offensive. Today, half of our nation is in shock and the other half in elation over last night's results. Leading up to that point, many fuels were set on fire via protests, offenses, split families and lost friendships. Ironically, Canada seems to be a more appropriate place to live as it was in 2008-2012. If your candidate didn't win, it's not the end of the world. America is still a great place to live when you can encounter those true loving souls who genuinely care. God is always in control.

Over the years, I have survived things that could have led me into bitterness, despair and depression. One case in point: Mom developed Alzheimer's disease and needed skilled care. I was in college at the time when the decision was made to place her in a facility. I disagreed, dropped everything and began caring for Mom at home for the next seven years. It was a labor of love with no physical ongoing help from family. There is a coping mechanism to every situation. I chose to love and forgive. However, some don't choose this path and later reap the consequences. In previous elections love and prayer was placed on the back burner. Let your fruit of love and patience manifest always under the severest of circumstances. Those who need healing are depending on it.

As the gloating, bitterness, finger-pointing and insensitive comments prevail, let your fruit of patience and love be the catalyst for extending the olive branch to our brothers and sisters. Now let's all sit down in God's classroom and learn the lesson He's teaching.

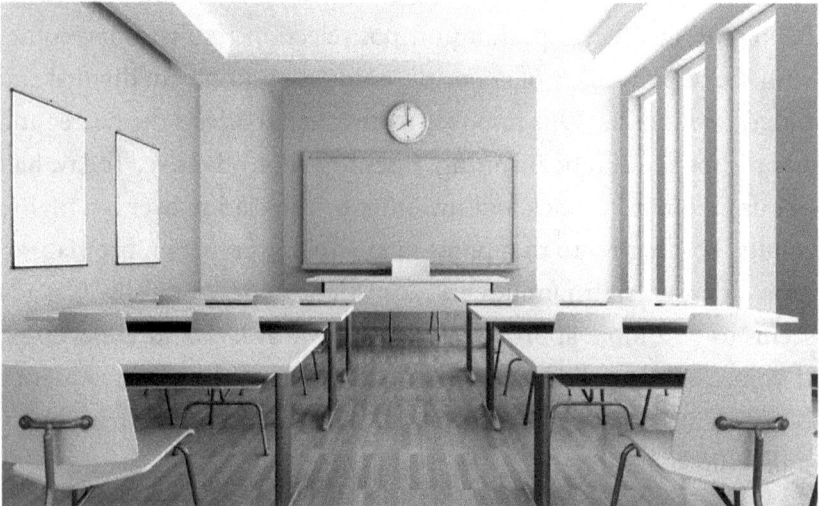

Let's Pray

Oh God! Tensions are high. Hearts are broken. So many lives are snuffed out on both sides. Let comfort reign over these families that have suffered loss in Dallas as well as across this nation. Let understanding and restraint take the place of agitation and fear. Stop the plan of Satan that is working in the minds of those who seek to further violence and bloodshed. Dispatch your angels to minister to and protect our citizens as well as law enforcement and other public officials. Help us to look for opportunities to show kindness and forgiveness in the midst of these tragedies, in the name of Jesus.

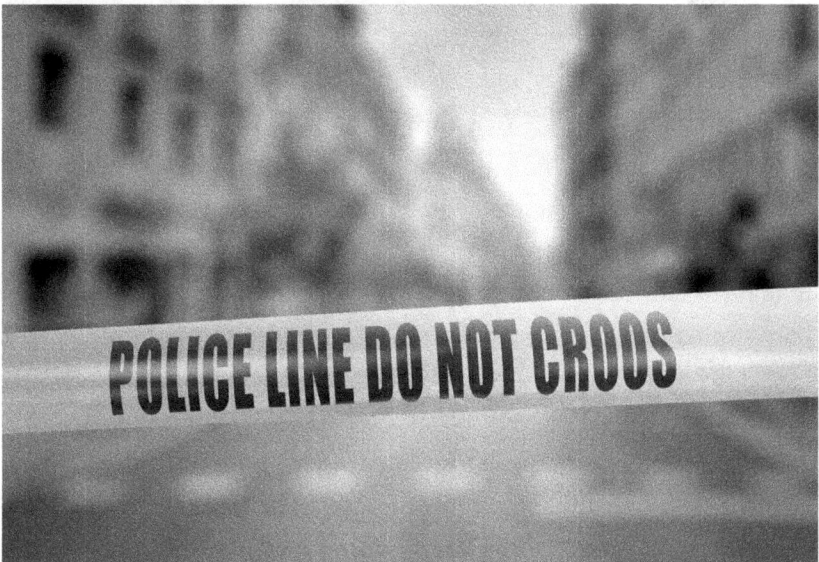

Let The Weak Say I Am Strong

We've heard that when a person is off their meds they may act out of character or, "God forbid," begin a path of destruction to themselves or others. The medication prescribed was producing a calming effect to prevent such action. Well, look out, saints! I'm off the prescribed medications. I've started out on a path of destruction! The damage is going to be lethal!

Persons diagnosed with cancer in most cases suffer more from the actual side effects of the medication prescribed. And the physicians say that benefits outweigh the negative effects, which can be managed. Only the patient can tell the story and decide whether quality of life or quantity of life is more important. When we walk this journey with the Lord, he knows the beginning from the end. We can trust him to decide what the end is going to be. Jesus took our infirmities and bore our sicknesses when he became our Lamb for the slaughter on the cross of Calvary. He took many stripes for our healing... I believe and trust in his word. While I'm waiting for God to perfect his plan in my life and fight my battles, I'm taking every opportunity to tell the good news that Jesus saves.

A child of God who is on this journey offers many sacrifices of praise (praising God in difficult circumstances). The activities of daily living, ADLs, such as walking or standing, are limited. The eyesight may be a little blurry, and pain may be constant. When God sends relief and strength, it is celebrated. When God gave me strength for the first time on this journey, I went out and cut the grass in the front yard with a huge weed eater. I was like a person who had not eaten in a week and finally got food. In this case, I had been without strength to even attempt anything like this in three years. I couldn't clean my house or even stand up in the kitchen to cook a meal.

Being off the meds is only destructive and lethal to Satan, the one who wants to keep us down. He was already defeated on the cross by Jesus. He is an illusionist and hopes that you are not reading the word of God that uncovers him. If you don't know Jesus, you are missing the benefits he has for those who love him. Take the time to repent and give him your heart today. Receive all that he has for you. He said in his word that in my weakness His strength is made perfect. Every bit of strength that God gives me is used against Satan. I can walk longer distances to tell people about Jesus, I can drive to church and praise him in the beauty of holiness, I can write about his goodness and encourage my brothers and sisters. Find what your hands and feet can do for the Lord. Trust him with your life. #redeemingthetime

Matthew 8:17; Isaiah 53:4-5; Psalm 27:14; 2 Chronicles 20:17; 2 Corinthians 12:9; St. John 3:3-7; John 3:16

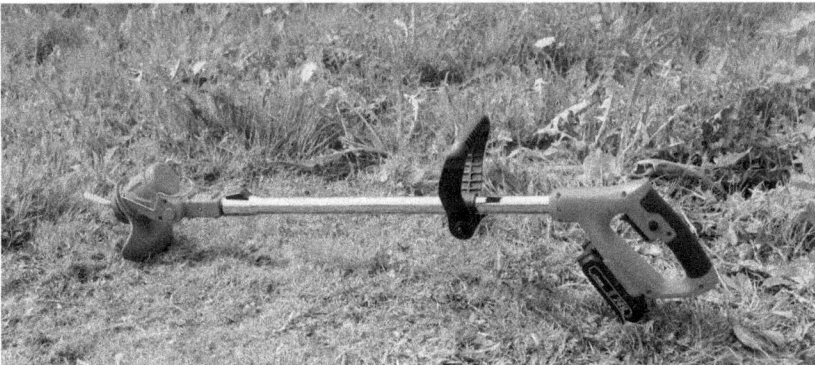

Look Up And See God

Look for the silver lining.

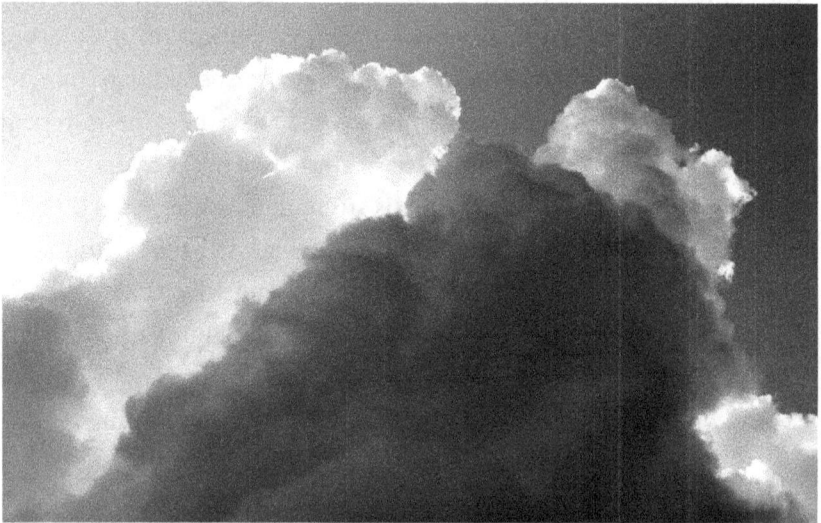

Love Is The Key

From Macrina Wiederkehr: While America figures this all out, I'm going to continue holding doors open for strangers, letting people cut in front of me in traffic, saying please and thank you, saying good morning, being patient with a waiter, and smiling at strangers as often as I am provided the opportunity. I will not stand by idly and let children live in a world where unconditional love is invisible. Join me in showing love and respect to those who may not necessarily seem to deserve it. Find your own way to swing the pendulum in the direction of love because today, sadly, hate seems to be winning. I want us to live in a world where hate has no place!

Positivity has to start somewhere, and love overpowers hate.

It is vital that we remember that we can disagree and still be respectful.

Copied and pasted this from a friend, who got it from another friend, who got it from another friend.

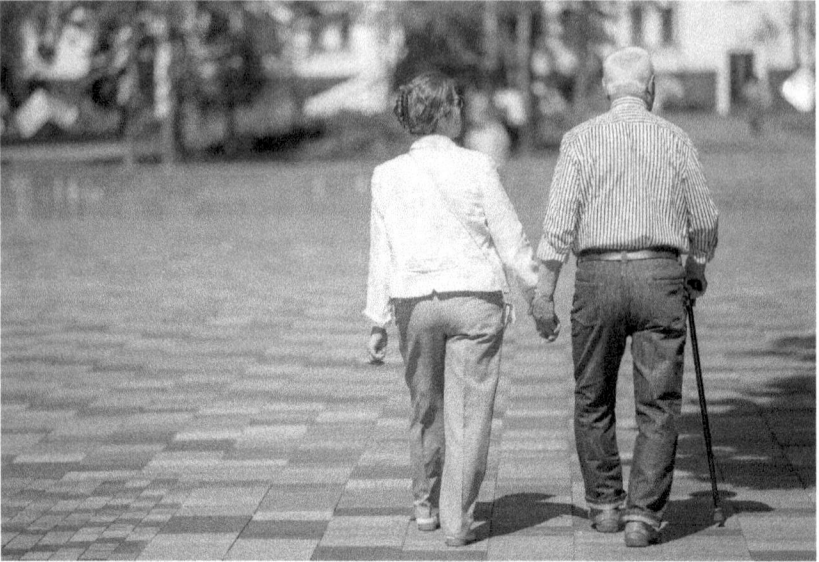

Love Lifted Me

As we try to put a padlock on disobedience and attempt to lock down sin with temporary legal fixes, Satan our adversary is having a field day dividing and conquering the masses. Social and political agendas have become wars of rhetoric far above cohesive understanding, in exchange for demonization of every cause, lifting up hate.

Too many are wearing the Scarlet Letter and walking on eggshells, wondering what to do at the polls and worrying about the mindset of unregenerate candidates. There was a popular outreach program called Scared Straight for incorrigible youth, designed to give them the experience of incarceration. After walking in the shoes of criminals for a day or two, many vowed never to do anything that would lead to incarceration.

I took the challenge of coming out of my comfort zone and went down into the trenches to experience the cure for complacency. There you will find the lost and unloved crying out for love and understanding. There you will find the masses who are not or refuse to be locked down by laws, who continue in sin. There are clinics in every neighborhood visited by women and girls waiting for someone to say in love that there is a better way to plan a family. There are foreigners, strangers in our land, looking for a kind word, a smile or helping hand, who feel like targets in the midst of all the hate rhetoric. There are people with identity issues who've never heard the truth in love. There you will find that God is pleased with our outreach and love for the lost and our desire to lift up the name of Jesus before a lost and dying world.

The most obvious revelation is that we were once in the trenches, "sinking deep in sin, far from the peaceful shore. Very deeply stained within, sinking to rise no more. But the Master of the sea heard our despairing cry." Through the lyrics of that old hymn "Love Lifted Me," I'm reminded that had it not been for Jesus I would still be in that same sinful condition. One of God's precious saints told me one day how much God loves me. "When nothing else could help, Love lifted me." Let us walk in love to those that are without. #redeemingthetime

John 3:16; Matthew 5:9

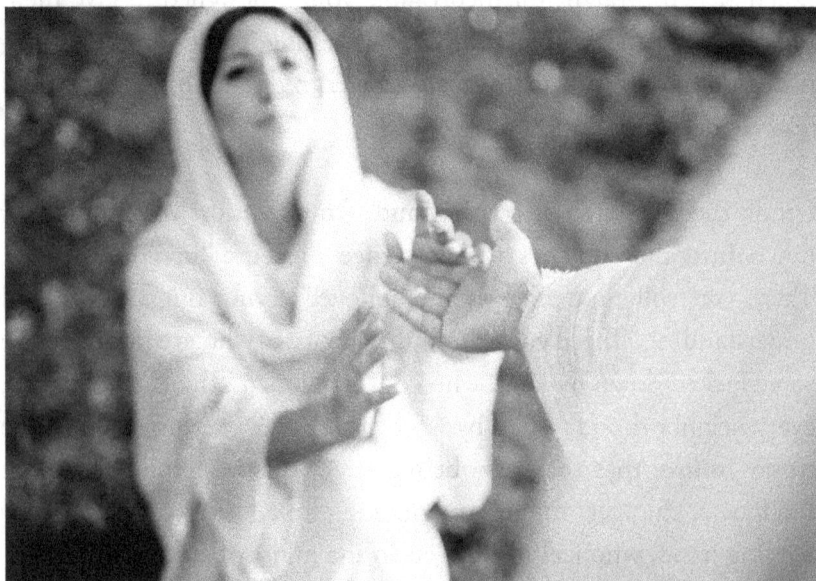

Make It Right

"Father, forgive them, for they know not what they do"—these are the words spoken by Jesus at His crucifixion. Who were they who were in need of God's forgiveness? In His last hour of temptation and suffering, the love of Jesus would be proclaimed down through the eons of time for His sacrifice in redeeming mankind back to God. Jesus forgave His torturers, who nailed His hands and feet to the cross. He asked forgiveness for the ones who put a crown of thorns on His head and pierced His side with a sword. His request to God included the religious leaders and soldiers who whipped, mocked, ridiculed and slandered Him. In spite of all He suffered before and during His trial, He remained humble.

When we truly realize the condition of our soul and submit to the will of God in receiving Jesus Christ as our Savior, we will receive help in living a righteous life. Talk to God every day in prayer and stay in His word. God is merciful and will help you grow through the trials and errors you encounter. Experience is the best teacher when applying the word of God to our lives. If you've been in the "WAY" forty years or more and still can't forgive your brother or sister and are still bound by things that don't please God, your soul is in trouble. Don't gamble with your soul another day but make it right with God. Don't put it off and let your tomorrows turn into days and weeks. #redeemingthetime

John 3:16; Luke 23:34; 1 Peter 2:22; 1 Peter 4:18-19; Proverbs 27:1;
Philippians 2:12

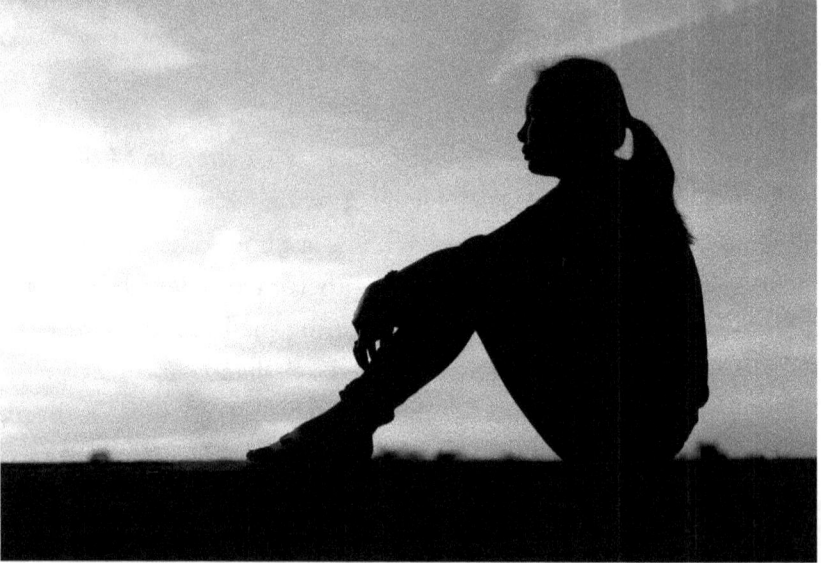

Make Me An Example

Each time I read the book of Acts I am humbled before the Lord. Stepping out of the "First century world" of the Apostles back into the 21st century is an eye-opener. My thoughts immediately focused on the current persecution of the church here and abroad. My prayers are always with the families of the beheaded, those who were mass murdered (by burning) in the churches and other atrocities for "not denying the Faith," and those who are remaining steadfast in the Lord. We have come a long way in exhibiting who Christ is and following after the pattern of the Apostles. Paul on many occasions reasoned in the synagogues every Sabbath and persuaded the Jews and the Greeks that Jesus was the Christ. God's power was with him in performing special miracles. The Word of God prevailed because of his obedience to the call of God. Paul suffered many insurrections (resistance) due to greed and pride. The officials didn't want to hear about a new King, and those who were saved discontinued their evil practices that normally brought a financial benefit for fortune telling.

Generating revenue in the 21st century brings about many hurtful lusts for many, as well as the church. It is overwhelming and challenging to deal with the many rules and regulations of this day and time associated with the same. God's grace is sufficient for these challenges, but many have failed. As a result, the church is seen as a money-making opportunity, only to generate ongoing revenue as the world does, competing with a capitalistic society. Paul was lied about and jailed, particularly for having an impact on the flow of revenue. He was beaten and put in stocks, but began to praise and worship the Lord in the midnight hour. God shook the foundation of the jail and loosed the bonds of all the prisoners. Paul preached, resulting in the head of security and his whole family being saved. He was later released and continued to preach Jesus throughout the regions.

The impact of lifting up Jesus is the salvation of souls. The impact of the salvation of souls is less evil, greed and pride, etc. The impact of following through on what God has commissioned the Christian to do is persecution. Apostle Paul reasoned with the people, brought deliverance to a fortune teller, performed miracles, praised God in the storm, and moved on from rebels to those who wanted to hear the Word. Whose pattern are you following? #redeemingthetime

Acts 16:16-40; Acts 18:4; Acts 18:12-16; Acts 19:11; Acts 19:18-20; 1Timothy 6:9-10; Acts 13:50-52; 2 Corinthians12:9

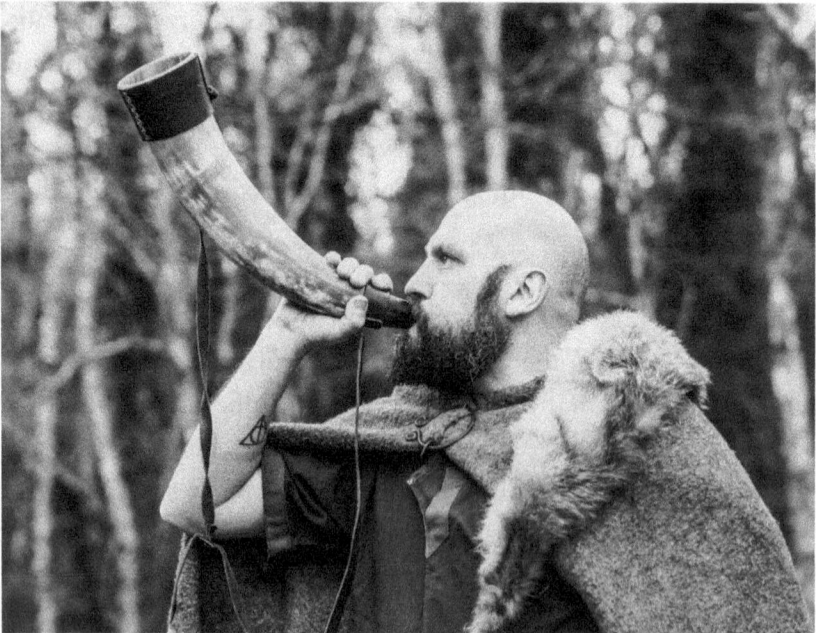

Make Me Over Lord

God told the Prophet Jeremiah to go down to the potter's house to hear his words. There he took clay and remade it over into another vessel. As the clay is in the potter's hand, so are we in God's hands. In this scenario, God was willing through Jeremiah to let all Israel know that he would reverse his judgments against them if only they would repent. They were admonished by God to return from their evil ways and make their ways and doings good. The people were burning their sons with fire for burnt offerings unto the idol Baal. It was called a horror, the blood of innocents, causing many who passed by to shake their heads. Instead of heeding God's warning and offer, the people plotted against Jeremiah. "Come, let us smite him with the tongue, and let us not give heed to any of his words." God is not pleased with naming his name and doing the opposite of his word for all the world to see. Jeremiah was hated for his strict criticism of priests, prophets, pastors and temple cults, who destroy and scatter the people of God.

In this age of grace and truth, sin and corruption should not once be named among clergy or those naming the name of Christ. No need to reveal the gory details. God has exposed many. If you have been a work in progress and in the "church hospital" for 42 years, it is now time for you heed God's call on your life and get up to help your brothers and sisters contend for the faith. God's grace is sufficient and not to be frustrated. His mercy and forgiveness is abundant.

When the governor, son of a priest of Israel, heard that Jeremiah prophesied their fate for disobedience, Jeremiah was beaten, jailed and put in stocks. History states that brave Jeremiah continued to speak for God, was spared death and escaped with the help of a eunuch. He was faithful until his death in Egypt. He was also transparent in that he had periods of despondency. But God's word was in Jeremiah's heart as a burning fire shut up in his bones. He testified, "I could not keep quiet." Is God molding you to be a Jeremiah? His grace is sufficient for you. #redeemingthetime

Jeremiah 18:1-2; Jer. 20:7-12; Jer. 23:1-2; Jer. Chapter 26; Galatians 2:21; Timothy 1:14

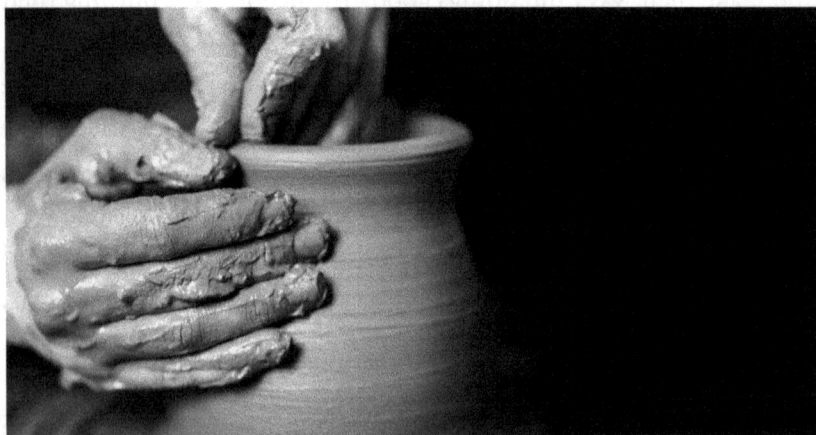

Merciful Father

I witnessed among many today a murder on national TV and social media—a murder of a Black man pleading for his life while being held down in the street by a nonchalant white police officer with his hand in his pocket, kneeling on the neck of the victim. I am grieved that he suffered without compassion for his pleading. My heart goes out to the family most likely traumatized by the way he died.

I left law enforcement in 1986 when as a supervisor in charge of a jail unit, I was told by my superior to change the details of an incident that happened there. I was instructed to remotely open the cell door and let the captain and his lieutenants inside. I observed them go in and assault an obviously unruly inmate. My report of the incident was detailed but not accepted by my superior. I resigned after being told to change it. I had to decide if I was going to be a part of the *old boy" network or maintain my integrity.

The lack of honesty and integrity in the upper ranks of protection and leadership is a problem. We have a lot of good officers mixed with bad eggs, where most never get thrown out.

My prayer for this incident and the many lives lost unjustly that preceded it is that the perpetrators be brought to justice. Images of this murder are forever etched in my mind. My own son, who was facing 60 years, was given 35 years for being in the wrong place at the wrong time for a murder involving a drug exchange. Although he's still claiming his innocence and working with the Innocence Project, the courtroom images of the deceased and descriptions of his death were too much to bear. God brought me through that valley.

Our black people are dying unjustly. If you are passionate and anxious about our plight, receive God's love and comfort while he sees that justice is served. #redeemingthetime.

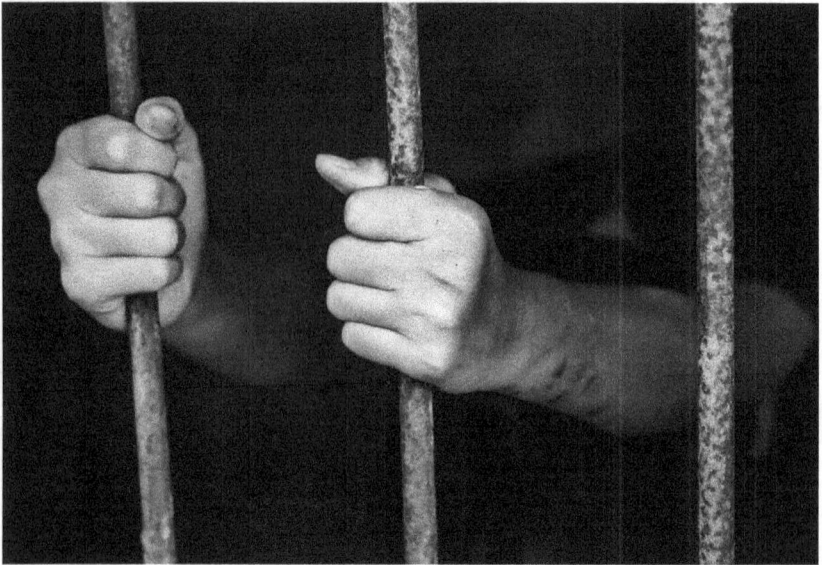

Mighty God

Our God sits on a sapphire throne. Imagine that. What could be more fitting than for the Almighty God, maker of the Universe, creator of mankind and judge of the world to sit on a throne of precious stone? The Bible speaks of crystal rivers, golden streets, gates of pearl, and mansions prepared for those who have kept the faith. It is written that eyes have not seen, ears have not heard, nor has it even entered into the heart of man the things that God has prepared for them who love him. My ancestors and those who loved the Lord were not allowed to read the Bible or other books and learn about life during slavery. They could not read and relied mostly on oral tradition; stories passed down from one generation to the next. They viewed their journey to Heaven, anticipating a "Cabin In The Sky" until the day they died. What a glorious day it will be when they see what has really been prepared for them. We are without excuse in denying a true and living God when we can look around and see the mighty works of God everywhere on earth. Everything that was ever made came from the earth. Our Creator, the Almighty God, is the Originator of everything. He gets the glory!

God has a plan for every man, woman, boy and girl born into this world. We don't have to wonder about it or wonder who God is. He sent us his love gift Jesus Christ in all of his mercy to redeem us back to him. In order to get to that beautiful place called Heaven, ask for forgiveness and receive Jesus Christ into your heart. "God so loved the world that he gave his only begotten son Jesus Christ, that whosoever believes on him should not perish but have everlasting life." #redeemingthetime

1 Corinthians 2:9; Romans 1:20; Revelations 22:1; Rev. 21:21; Ezekiel 1:26; John 3:16; John 14:2-3

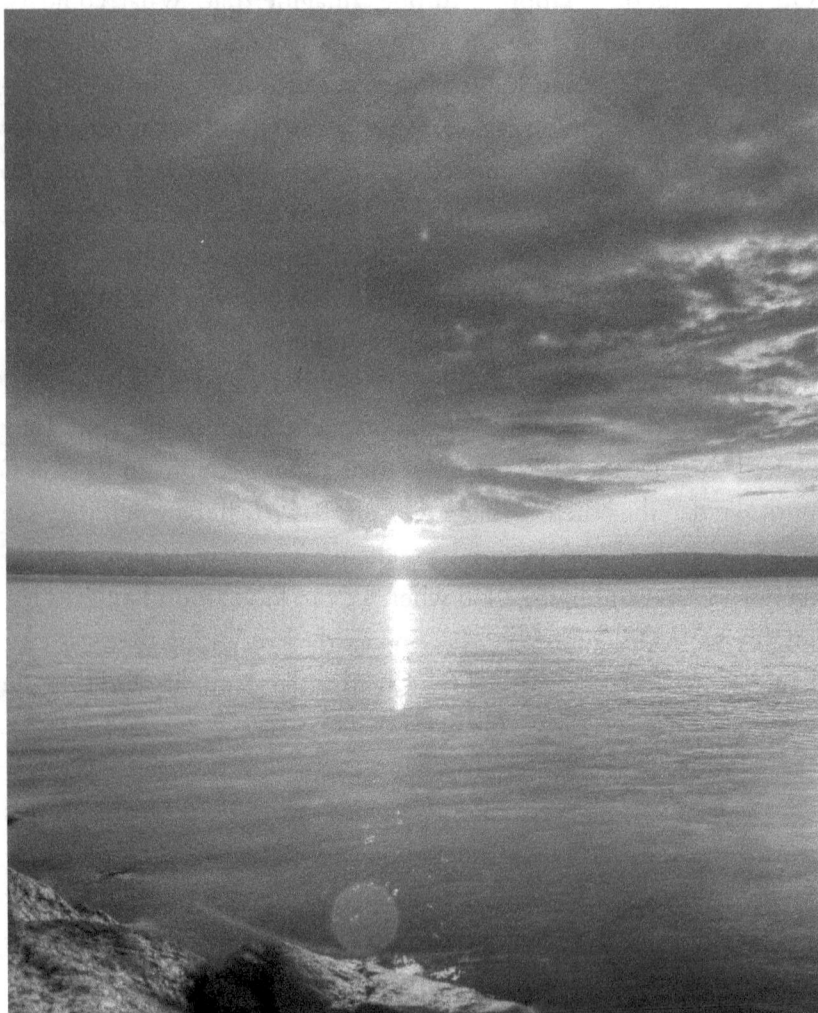

Moments In Time

There is something called "white noise." To those who are familiar with it, no doubt they've learned that it's a welcomed moment in time and a benefit while convalescing.

As the days pass by, I find myself occupying and embracing what we most take for granted. The wind and rain were blowing the other night and the sound of it sweeping across the window gave thought to my peace and safety. The continuous noise from the storm's effect upon the window created a tranquil mood of pleasant calmness. Those who are hospitalized have the opportunity to switch to a TV channel that offers white noise. It's the auditory experience of sound that lacks musical quality. Among its many benefits and technical uses, patients in hospitals enjoy relaxation and peaceful rest from the same.

Whether it's man-made white noise or nature's peaceful attractions, it is a space in time I have reserved to listen for God's voice. Sometimes when we think God will answer in some spectacular way, He catches us off guard and speaks in a "still small voice." Embrace your peaceful moments and listen for the gentle voice of God. #redeemingthetime

1 Kings 19:11-13

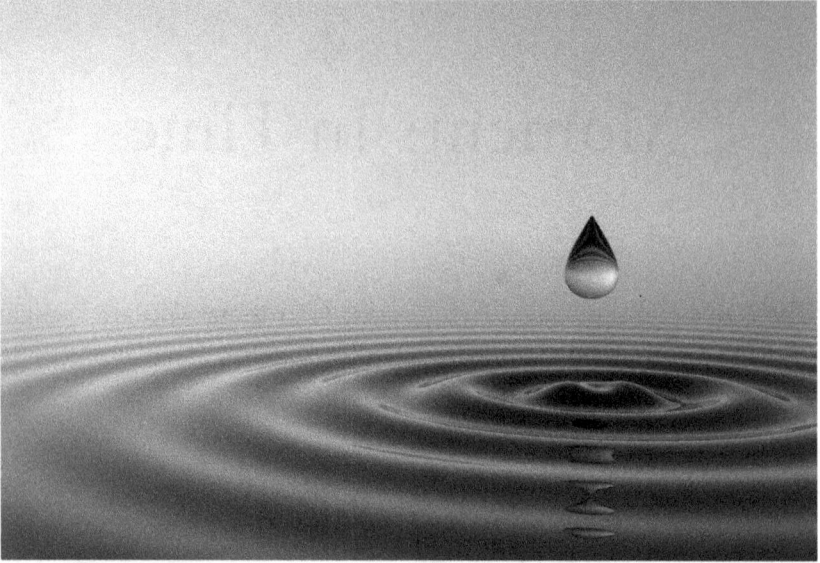

What's Important?

Anyone who knows Kyrzayda Rodriguez the famous fashion blogger knows she died right after announcing she had Stage 4 stomach cancer. These were her words on her last days on earth. May her soul rest in peace.

"I have a brand-new car parked outside that can't do anything for me. I have all kinds of designer's clothes, shoes and bags that can't do anything for me. I have money in my account that can't do anything for me. I have a big well-furnished house that can't do anything for me.

Look, I'm lying here in a twin-size hospital bed. I can take a plane any day of the week if I like, but that can't do anything for me.

So do not let anyone make you feel bad for the things you don't have. The things you have, be happy with those. If you have a roof over your head, who cares what kind of furniture is in it? The most important thing in life is LOVE.

Lastly, make sure you enjoy the ones you love.

See, in life anything you have—material things, possessions, riches, fame can't do anything for you once you leave this earth.

Let God be the reason for our existence. Only what you do for Christ will last. #redeemingthetime

National Day Of Prayer

On this day that has been set aside as a National Day of Prayer, oh God, my heart is heavy. Come and see about us all, oh God, who were born into the world and those who are waiting to be born. Look upon us now, oh God, and let your hand of mercy be stretched out still. Some of us know You and Your plan for our lives. Many of us have yet to find You and come to know You in the pardon of our sins. Have mercy upon those who oppose You and Your plan for all mankind. Help us to see that Jesus Christ paid a great price for our souls to be redeemed back to You.

Touch the heart that's hard against Your will. Open the eyes of our leaders of this great nation to see the truth of Your Word, that it may be applied to every important decision rendered. Have mercy on the suffering Christians and their families that are being persecuted and killed. Oh God, we know that no man can come to You except through Jesus Christ, Your love gift to the world. As Your people continue to lift up Jesus before the world, draw the hearts to You. Jesus said, "If I be lifted up I will draw all men unto me." Come see about us, dear God. Save the children and babies that are in harm's way, in the name of Jesus.

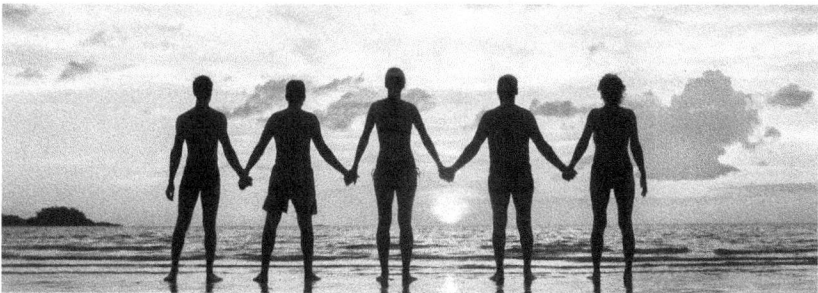

New Strength

I had a glorious weekend in the Lord feasting on the Word of God, fellowshipping with the Saints, and participating in the Blood Cancer Awareness Walk-A-Thon. Because I was not able to walk the distance, I rented a transport chair for the occasion. Yesterday, for the first time in three years since a diagnosis of Multiple Myeloma Bone Cancer, I was able to run up the stairs and back down, walk around my block and take out the trash with no shortness of breath.

GOD HAS GIVEN ME NEW STRENGTH! I was at Pep Boys getting my car serviced yesterday when I noticed a difference physically. When I got home and found that I could run up and down the stairs I immediately began to praise the Lord for his faithfulness to His Word and for always being available to hear the cries of the righteous. Jesus took our infirmities and bore our sickness. Matthew 8:17. I first testified to my family because they knew personally what the struggle had been and now, they also gave God Praise. I'm thanking everyone who has prayed and has been with me on this journey. Please continue. God is faithful to His Word and will also hear your cry of repentance. Give him your heart today.

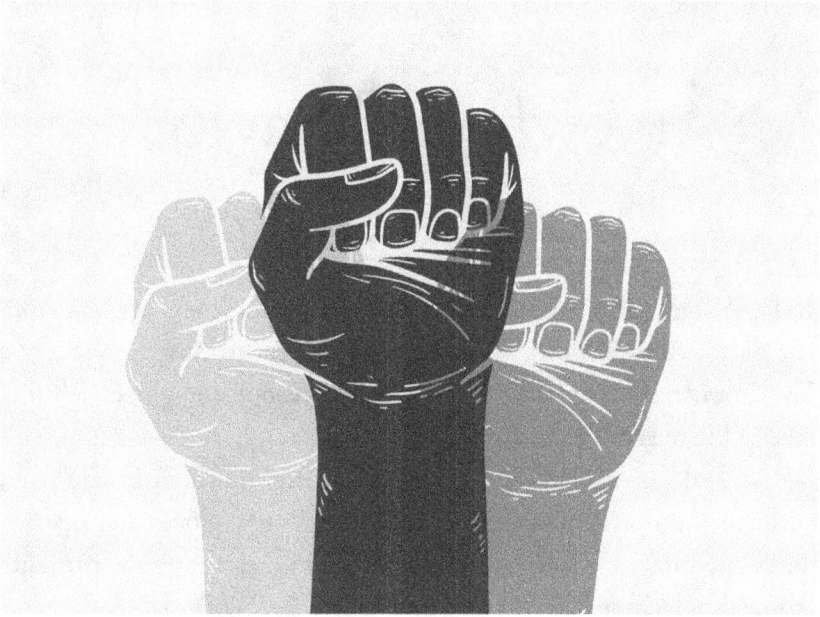

Newfound Savior

Easter Sunday 1955: I remember the smell of newness coming from the Easter clothes Mom had bought us to wear to church. She tied a bow in my head that had a matching pocketbook and gloves. All that week I looked for "Peter Cottontail," who sang Easter was on its way. We looked forward to coloring eggs and hiding them in the front yard for a hunt. I must have examined my new gloves and opened and closed my new pocketbook a hundred times before the preacher stopped preaching.

Thus began my understanding of Easter to include gobbling down pink and yellow marshmallow chicks all week. I grew up hoping to be a part of the Easter Parade held annually in downtown Baltimore. Finally, at the age of 17, I went out and bought a hot pink hat, hot pink gloves, hot pink cape and hot pink shoes. I was on my way to the Easter Parade. Nobody could tell me I didn't look good walking down Pennsylvania Avenue.

Who knew that six years later I would come to know the true meaning of Easter? I received Jesus Christ into my heart in 1972. "For God so loved the world that He gave His only begotten Son that whosoever believes in Him should not perish but have everlasting life." Had He not been crucified, buried and rose on the third day, my mind would still be blinded to the real meaning of Easter. Give Jesus your heart this Easter Sunday. #redeemingthetime

St John 3:16; 1 Corinthians 15:3-4

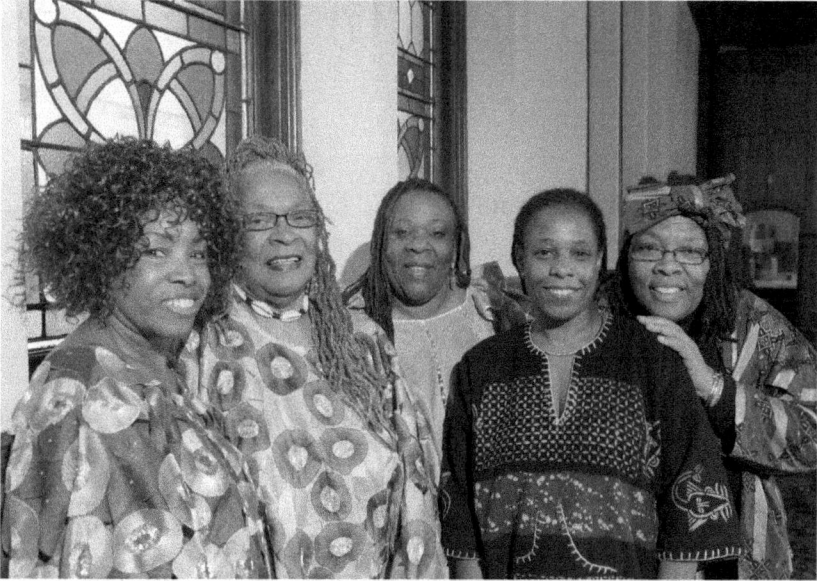

No Fear In Love

As I lay here recovering from a Carotid Endarterectomy, nursing pain and a wound made to my neck, I am at the same time thanking all who prayed and giving God the glory for bringing me through this surgery. Our adversary Satan would have us fearful, doubtful and with a whole lot of "what-ifs." Satan is a defeated foe! Jesus Christ gave his life on the cross of Calvary to destroy the works of Satan and to redeem us back to God. Satan knows the Word of God and is counting on you to forget it and not use it against him. True Christians don't have to fear. There is no fear in love. Perfect love casts out all fear. I went into surgery trusting in his Word, knowing that he is with me in whatever situation I encounter.

Christians have authority over Satan. The immutable, never-changing Word and the prayers of the Saints run him right out of town to plan his next attack. Be prepared. Trust God and stay in his Word. #redeemingthetime.

1 John 3:8; 1 John 4:18; Luke 10:17-19; James 5:15; 2 Timothy 2:15

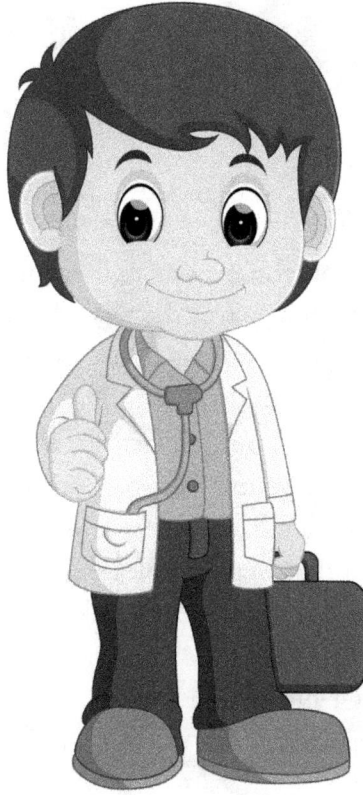

No Regrets

Living with regrets? Tonight, prayers and encouragement went up for a sister in the Lord from across the seas. She is one of many who have taken advantage of the online group Global Media Outreach, which ministers to those worldwide coming to the Internet looking for God. Her progress bears out the fact that she loves the Lord and wants to please him. As a young Christian, she found herself caught up in a deception via family members and succumbing to activities (more than once) that were not pleasing to God. She wrote via email requesting prayer over her regret, asking for courage to cease the activity. "Please do kindly pray with me. I really need help; I am really regretting that I did such a thing." Here is the response via encouragement and prayer:

You have a healthy conscience. There are many in the Bible who God loved that had to live with regrets. King David was a man after God's own heart who plotted to obtain another man's wife. He repented with Godly sorrow and remained to become the one to fulfill all of God's will (2 Samuel Chapter 11; 1 Samuel 13: 14; Acts 13:22). Rahab the harlot's life was spared along with all of her family because she helped the servants of God fulfill God's plan for his people Israel. She remained with the people of God for the rest of her days (Joshua 6: 25; James 2:25). Rahab was mentioned in the genealogy of Jesus Christ. What an honor!

God said though your sins be as scarlet he will make them white as snow (Isaiah 1:18)! Acknowledge your sin to God today and ask for forgiveness. Don't put it off any longer. He is faithful and just to forgive us of all unrighteousness (1 John 1:9). The tests of our hearts only come to show us those things lurking in us that do not please God.

Father, touch my sister today with your love. Give her renewed strength and courage to make the right decision concerning this matter at hand. Heal her heart that she may move forward in righteousness to put you first in her life, in the name of Jesus. Let the love of God heal your regrets today. Turn them all over to him and make Jesus Christ the Lord of your life. #redeemingthetime

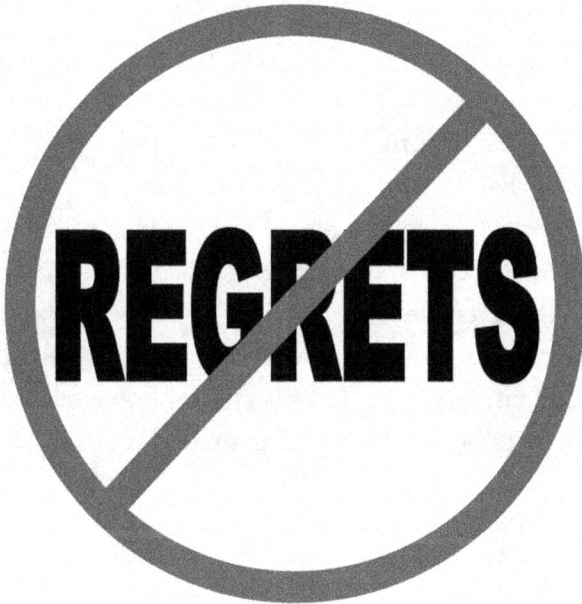

Others May But You Cannot

There is a lot going on that shocks my conscience as a Christian, and there are several ways that I address issues to help generate solutions. I am thoroughly convinced that on-going arguments and rants have their place, but to the disadvantage of some. Those "some" are walking around on eggshells afraid to disagree, have been badly injured or have died because of disagreements. The words we choose to speak or "agree with" and how we speak those words, particularly on various "hot button issues" may be fueling a fire in the mind of the unstable.

That may be stretching the point a bit, but it doesn't take a rocket scientist to see that the world is tense, fearful and on edge. People just want to know that somebody cares enough to look past the faults and show genuine concern. When things get bad enough, I want to be that person that's remembered as one who can get a prayer through, not as the one who stripped you of your dignity, dismantled your cause, or condemned you to Hell with words. Some call it, "righteous indignation." I call it, lack of wisdom. #redeemingthetime

John 3:17:18, Proverbs 11:30 - 31

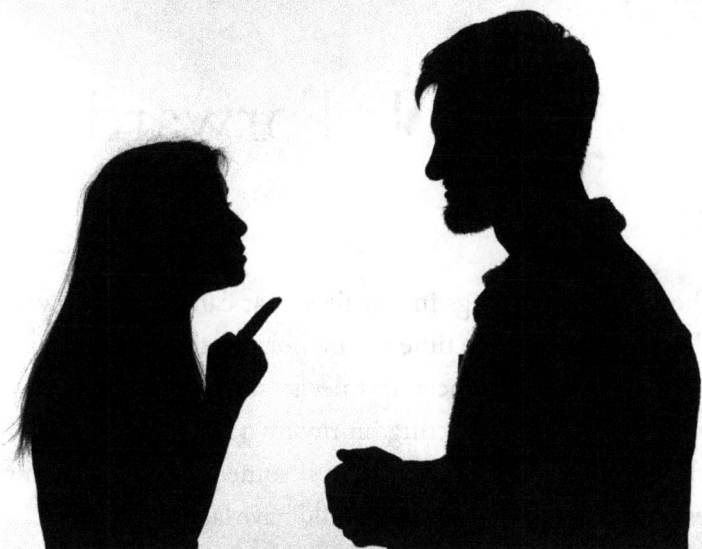

Pay It Forward

There are many things in our lives that can get in the way of God's plan for us. From the time we are born until we truly come to know God, our life experiences and decisions draw us closer to or farther away from Him. Reflecting on my own experiences, I often wonder where my life would have ended if someone had not told me about Jesus and his love. I guess you could have labeled me as RELIGIOUS, a faithful church member and worker on Sunday. I loved to dance and smoked two packs of Kools a day. We used to sing a song in church called "Holy Spirit, Don't Leave Me," which was an upbeat tune describing Jesus's temptation in the wilderness with Satan. I enjoyed the tune and the beat, but I didn't know Jesus or the Holy Spirit. The frame of mind I was in at that time is similar to many today whose minds are darkened to the truth of God and his plan.

I am grateful for the brave, committed saints of God who are working every day in every way to change the minds of the masses that are blind to the truth. Jesus said he didn't come into the world to condemn the world, but that the world through Him might be saved. I received the witness and believed on him in 1972, because someone was faithful to their commission and calling in the Lord. I'm paying it forward. #redeemingthetime

2 Corinthians 4:3-4; John 3:16 -17

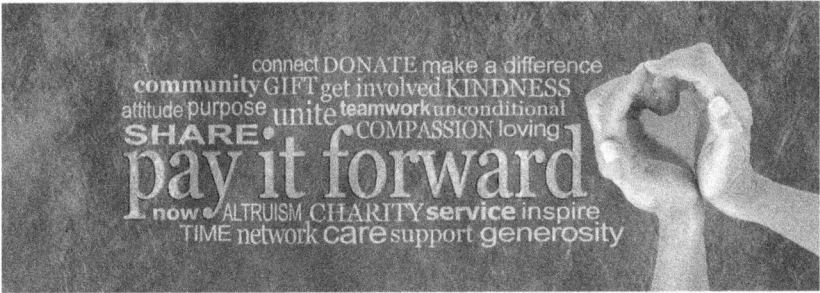

connect DONATE make a difference
community GIFT get involved KINDNESS
attitude purpose unite teamwork unconditional
SHARE COMPASSION loving
pay it forward
now ALTRUISM CHARITY service inspire
TIME network care support generosity

The Power Of God

Had audience today with THE ALMIGHTY GOD who sits on the GREAT WHITE THRONE, whose head and hair are white like wool and white as snow, whose eyes are like flames of fire. He is my strong tower where I run for safety and protection. My petition was made known to Him via my Savior Jesus Christ, who redeemed my soul back to God forty-seven years ago.

The presence of God was mighty in the sanctuary from many giving honor and praise due to our Lord. There was unity as hearts, minds and petitions reached God's throne. The windows of Heaven were opened. Our beings were gripped by God's presence, letting us know He is listening and concerned. Yes, He is concerned for the lost, those who are cast aside, the discarded, the sick, the backslider, the good, the bad and yes, even the ugly.

Weep, saints of God. Each time you shed a tear, a soul is drawn closer to and even born of God. When you pray and travail before the Lord, the scales fall off the eyes of those crying out silently in their soul for help. #redeemingthetime

Revelation 1:14; Proverbs 18:10; 1 Peter 5:8; Hebrews 9:15; Malachi 3:10; Hebrews 8:1; Romans 5:6; Proverbs 15:29; Luke 15:3-7; Joel 2:17

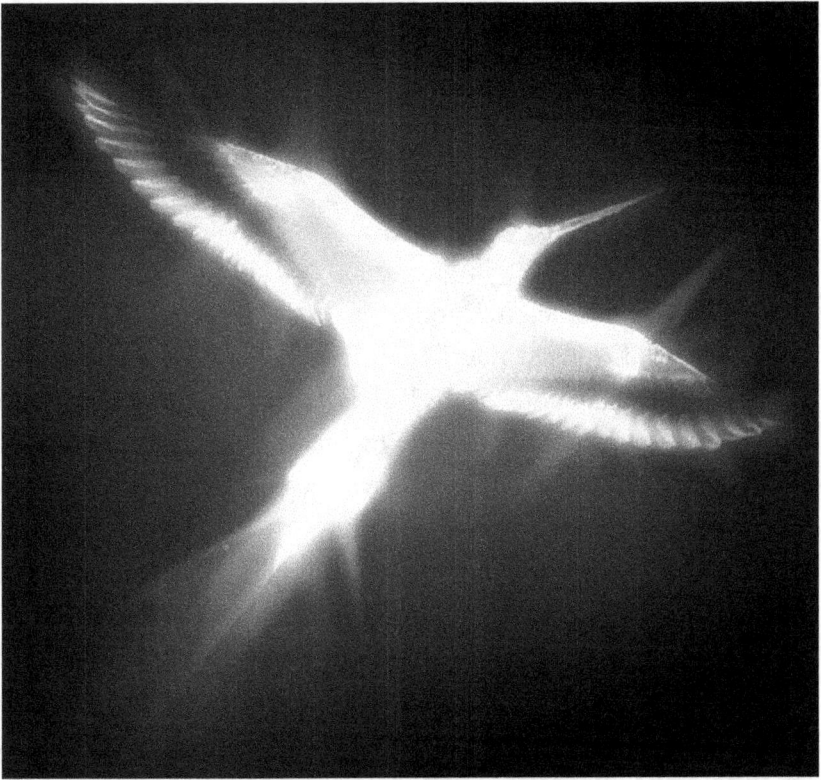

Praise Him In The Test

Getting to and from church today was a challenge but it was well worth it. David suffered many trials in his lifetime and spoke specifically about many of them. In Psalm 77 David appears upset with God at some point in his trial. He became overwhelmed, depressed and even despondent. God loved David in spite of his shortcomings and only wanted the best for him.

Like David, sometimes we wonder when God will bring us out of our situations that seem too hard to bear. We begin to question God. David asked, "Where is your mercy? Have you forgotten to be gracious?" When David began to remember the works of the Lord, he began to praise Him for His goodness and talk of His mighty, wonderful works. Soon there was no more room for complaints. When David began to change his way of thinking, he could then see light at the end of the tunnel. When in a test, change your way of thinking. Remember the works of the Lord in your own life, meditate on his goodness, talk of his mighty wonderful works, and Praise Him in the test. #togodbetheglory!

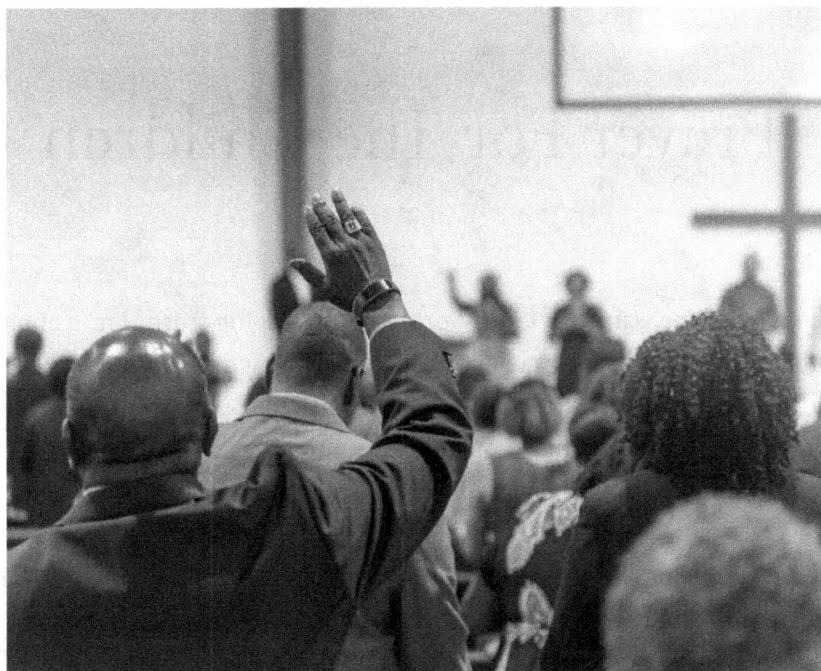

Prayer For The Children

Pray with me, saints of God. Lord, still this raging storm I'm feeling right now. Little children have been gunned down in Townville, S.C. Have mercy on the little children, Jesus. They haven't lived to know and understand life and to make their significant contribution. Jesus, come and see about us here on earth. It's bad, Lord.

Lives are being lost everywhere due to violence. I am fed up with the adversary and his works. My heart and soul is bothered daily by these tragedies here and throughout the world. Save the children out of harm's way, Lord. Send help and extend your hand of mercy. Jesus, Jesus, Jesus!

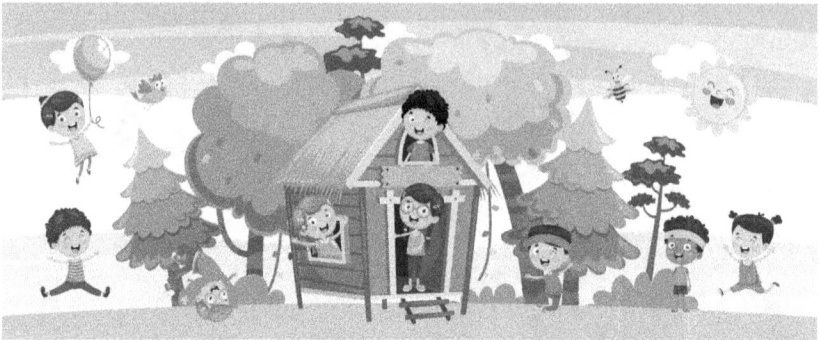

Prepared For God's Work

Oh my God! Oh my God! Heaven came down and the Glory of God filled the sanctuary. He blessed us in the praise and worship with a visitation of His power and anointing. This was a special time of God's refreshing to the Saints of God. Peter describes it in the Word of God as joy unspeakable and full of glory. When His presence fell in the sanctuary, I could no longer speak. Engulfed in His presence, as I felt His closeness, the tears of joy began to flow. I can't describe all that was happening to me, except that I experienced a touch of Heaven, and I did not want it to end.

However, we all have to come down to earth sometime and do the work that God called us to do as Christians. Therefore, I am refreshed one more time to shed the love of God abroad. Hunger and thirst after righteousness to experience these times of refreshing more often. Talk to God in prayer every day. Study God's Word. He's counting on us to be good representatives of His Word and His righteousness in a world that's calling good evil and evil good. #redeemingthetime

Psalm 63:2; 1 Peter 1:8; Acts 3:19; Nehemiah 8:10; Matthew 5:6; 2 Timothy 2:15; 1 Thessalonians 5:17; Romans 14:16-19; 2 Timothy 3:1-7

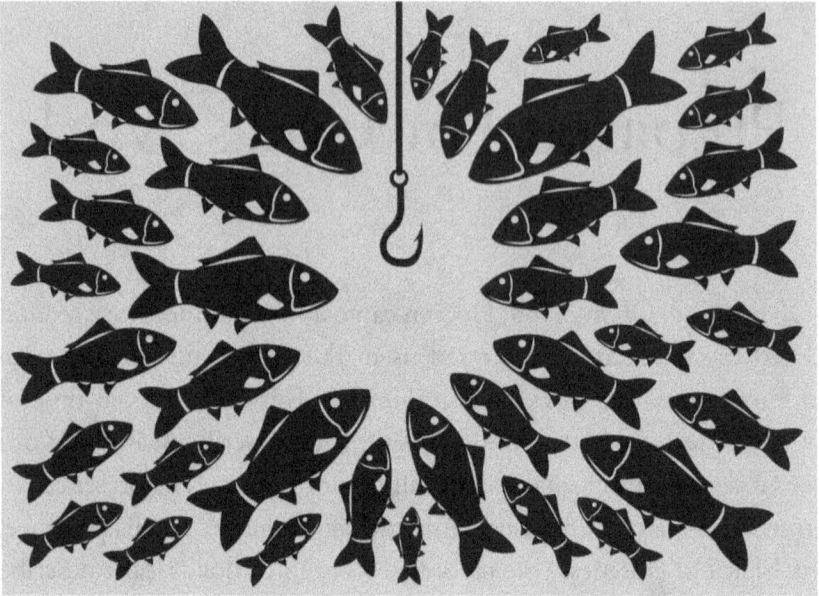

Reach Out And Touch

About 45 years ago I was standing on the corner waiting for the bus and feeling pretty bad about myself. I was in a backslidden state and out of the will of God. I saw two sisters from the church who seemed to recognize me. My heart started racing in anticipation, hoping they would come and say, "We miss you; come on back to church." But they just looked and whispered to each other as I boarded the bus. I remember thinking, *I guess I'm not good enough to get back to God*. But thanks be unto God, He reached down and picked me up, restored me, and wrapped His loving arms around me! REACH OUT TO SOMEONE TODAY and every day throughout the year. Souls are crying out anonymously, looking for God.

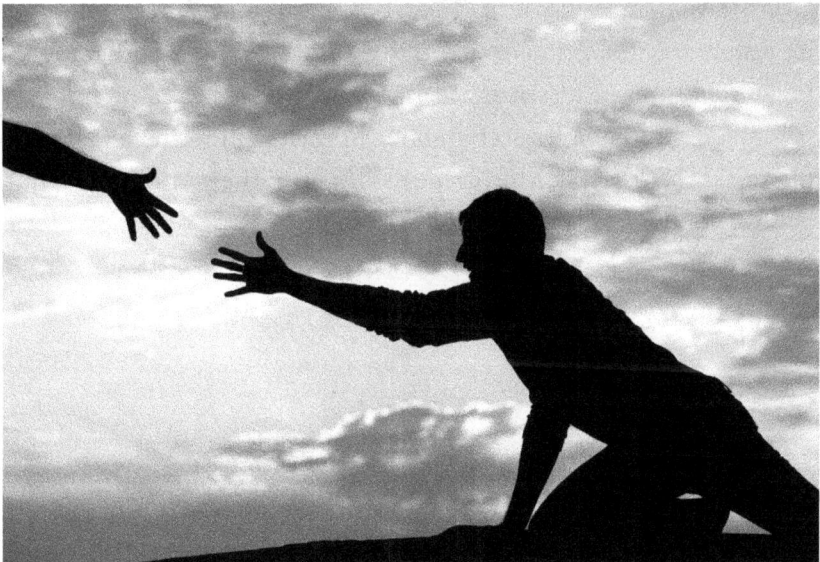

Reap The Harvest

There is a treasure that Christians have in their "earthen vessels." Many times, we feel the refreshing and manifestations of God's power in our places of worship. The power of God is also available to break yokes wherever we go. Somebody can be healed today, somebody can be strengthened today, and somebody can be saved today. We must be prepared every day to use that power and calling that God has given us to bring life. Study the Word daily to be able to provide an answer for the hope that is in you and to minister effectively to the lost. Pray in the spirit, talk to God and open the windows of Heaven with your petitions.

This excellent power is from God and not from us. Take care of it. Don't leave home without it. Take it to the grocery store, your favorite restaurant, the gym, school, work, your neighborhood and even to church. In the midst of all the issues and evil that're upon us, there is someone who's hoping, crying out in their soul for relief, and trying to rid themselves of the emptiness inside. The world is a harvest, and we are the reapers. #redeemingthetime

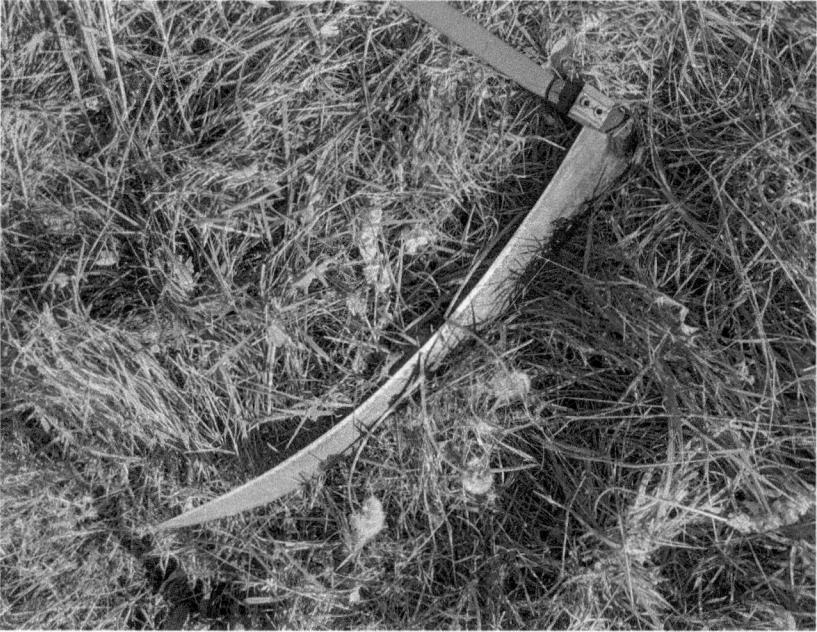

Reason To Prepare

My heart and prayers go out to families everywhere who have lost loved ones under tragic circumstances. I wonder what those people in Paris were thinking when they came face to face with the possibility of death. That would be a hard question to answer without first hearing their testimony. I am sure there are varying stories among those who survived not just this atrocity, but the many tragedies that are happening all over the world. It's not hard to imagine what they were "not thinking of " when faced with their own mortality. Most would be calling on the Lord for help. I pray that those who didn't survive were prepared to meet God.

A portion of my prayer each day is that the Lord would extend his hand of mercy to the lost; that they would have another opportunity to prepare for eternity. With the possibility of facing our own mortality, there are consolation and comforting words from our Lord and Savior Jesus Christ. "For God so loved the world that he gave his only begotten Son, that whosoever believes in him should not perish, but have everlasting life. For God sent not his Son into the world to condemn the world, but that the world through him might be saved." Give your heart to the Lord today. #redeemingthetime

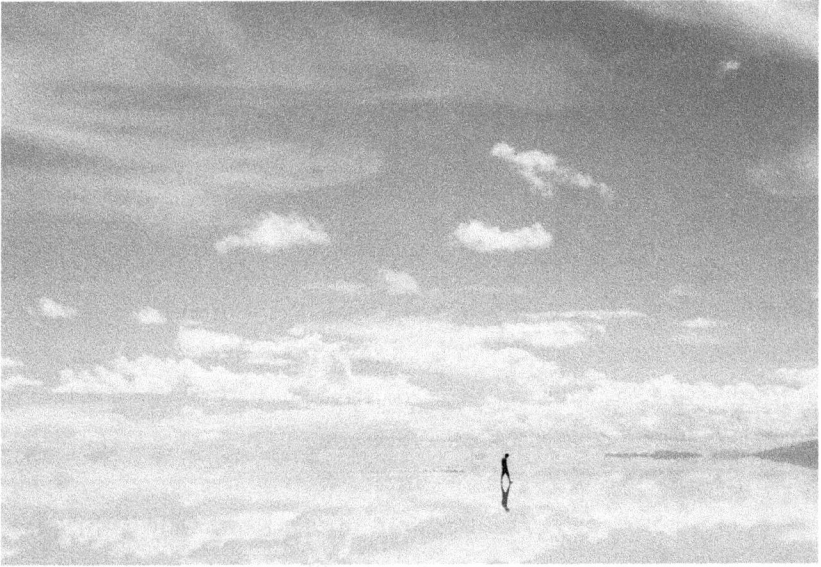

Refuge

Our God is a refuge and a fortress. I can go to him and feel peace and safety. There is a place in God for the righteous that the scriptures describe as secret—a place that is engulfed by the shadow of the Almighty God. It is a place where you can be covered completely with the presence of God all around, sweeping over your being like the warmth of a bath towel fresh out of the dryer. Why is this place called secret? It is unknown to others and unseen by others unless you dwell there, unless you have made up your mind to reside and settle in the presence of the Almighty God.

Our Most High God connects with us in this secret place with a little touch of Heaven and a strong desire to remain forever in his presence. Your soul and spirit feel right at home as God receives your praise and prayers, being touched by all that you are going through. One Sunday morning God's presence was mighty in the sanctuary after a soul-stirring message that touched my heart. The sanctuary was full and buzzing with conversation as the service ended. As I went right into prayer where I was seated, I could feel my spirit being lifted to another place that made the buzz and conversations seem a distance away. It was just me and God talking, without the distractions, in the secret place.

In God's fortress and tower there is safety, security and refuge. Dwelling in the secret place of the Almighty God gets God's attention.

Commit to keeping his attention by dwelling in the secret place every day. #redeemingthetime

Psalm 91:1-4; Proverbs 18:10

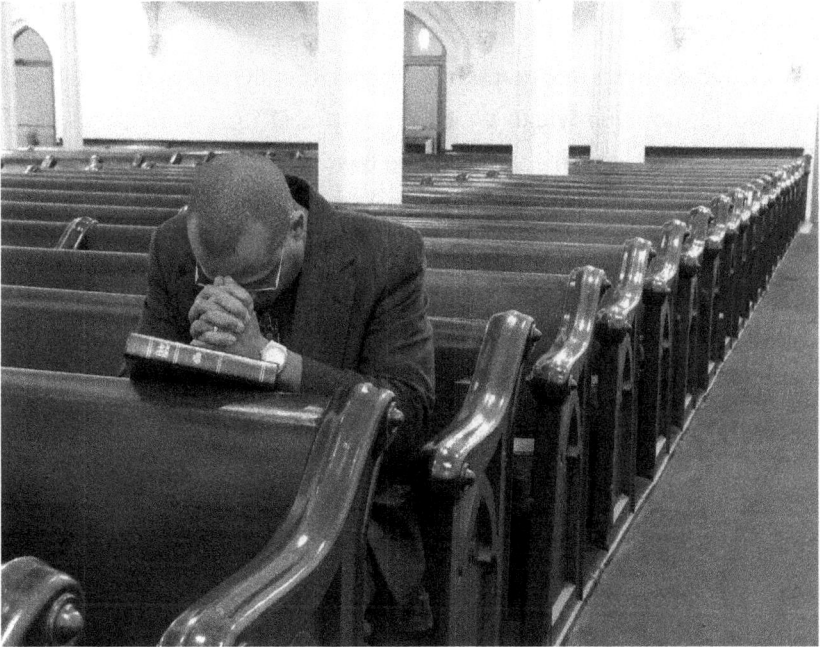

Seize The Opportunity

Now that we are all done taking a stand and sharing our ideals with the world, how many can we get to help heal the collateral damage? This is a good time to show that we have not compromised our witness as Christians who should be loving one another and showing love to all people.

The harvest is ripe, right here on social media. Just pick a topic surrounding the election outcome and you will find out how the world views us as Christians. In the midst of all the rhetoric and conversation, I have found hearts who really want to know the truth and gain understanding of it all. Therefore, it brings about an open door to a good witness in love. If you are up for this challenge, just hit on the topic of conversation and the section at the end to join the discussion. There you will find a world of conversation waiting for the manifestation of the sons of God. #redeemingthetime

Proverbs 11:30; Romans 8:21-22

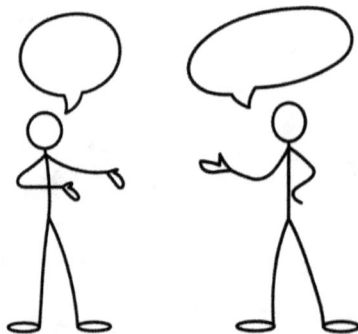

Seize The Victory

Ezekiel the Priest was sitting by a river when suddenly the heavens opened up and he saw visions of God. While being held in captivity by the current king under a heathen government, Ezekiel was chosen by God to prophetically speak to and warn his people about things to come. The visions were so grandiose, magnificent and astonishing that Ezekiel fell on his face in the presence of the glory of God. He heard the voice of the Lord coming from the vision of the likeness of a man sitting on a throne of sapphire surrounded by brightness, enfolding fire and rainbows.

Although Ezekiel was in exile, he was at peace. In our most severe trials, we can be at peace when we grow to recognize the devices of Satan against us. He will come hovering over us with negativity— huffing, puffing, threatening—trying to spoil our victory. Remind him of this: "Vengeance is mine saith the Lord. I will repay. Most likely Ezekiel was enjoying the peaceful, calm serenity of the river while meditating upon God. I don't believe he was complaining or shaking his fist at God for his dilemma. God spoke to him in his peaceful state of mind.

When you feel like you've had enough and just want to throw your hands up and quit, be reminded of God's word: "Be not overcome of evil, but overcome evil with good." (Romans 12:21, KJV) Let God speak to your spirit while in a peaceful state during the test, the trial, the exile, the captivity of your victory by Satan. Realize that the God of the Universe comes to your aid in the most severe temptations. He will repay. Visualize Him as Ezekiel did and seize the VICTORY!! #redeemingthetime

Ezekiel Chapter 1; Romans 12:19 – 20; Colossians 3:15

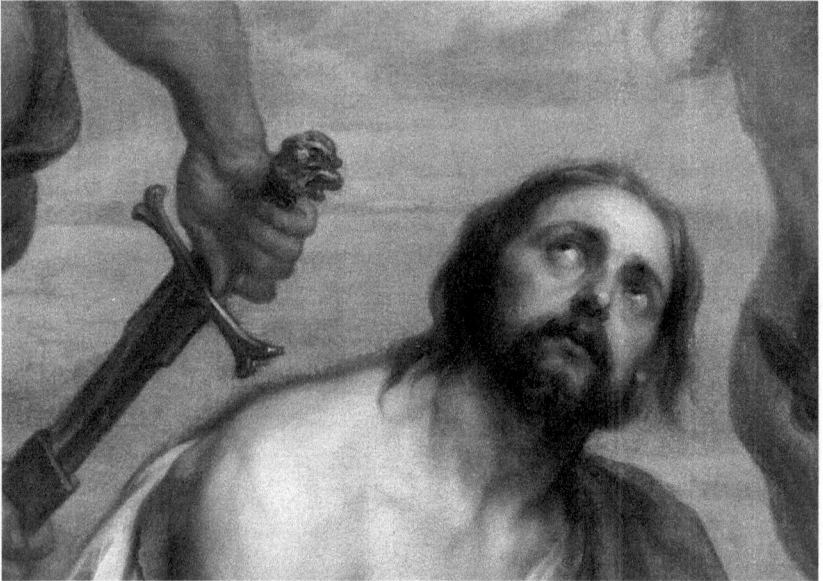

God-Inspired Unity

A message was preached in honor of Black History Month this Sunday. William J. Seymour and Lucy Farrow were featured as two African American ministers who impacted the Holiness Movement and the outpouring of the Holy Spirit on racism. They played an integral part in the return of Pentecostalism after years of spiritual drought.

Lucy Farrow received the baptism of the Holy Spirit with the evidence of speaking in tongues and provided the initial spark of revival. As the niece of abolitionist, orator, writer and statesman Frederick Douglass, Farrow began laying hands on people to receive the Holy Spirit.

In the face of adversity, oppression and frivolous Jim Crow laws, William J. Seymour, a praying man, began revival fires at 312 Azusa Street Mission in Los Angeles, CA. Seymour's connection to Farrow and Caucasian Methodist Pastor Charles Parham caused more than 10,000 people, black and white, to receive the gospel message, with many receiving the baptism of the Holy Spirit. "They exhibited racial harmony when America was racially divided. They were examples of what God can do to humbled hearts yielded to him." Eyewitness accounts testified, "The color line has been washed away in the blood of Jesus."

UNITY AND A HUNGER AND THIRST FOR GOD ARE
NEEDED IN THE BODY OF CHRIST.

1 Corinthians 1:26-31; Acts 1:8; Acts 2:42; Pastor Sharon Hardy
Knotts

A Day In Small Town. Usa....

...started with a parade in a town called Preston, celebrating school achievements, community efforts and lots of treats thrown to the laid-back, friendly residents who lined the streets at 10:00 a.m. There was no twirling, twerking or pelvic thrusts for little innocent eyes to wonder at this town where everybody seemed to know everybody. A special hometown air full of simple smiles and waves invited this friendly stranger to stay a little longer. On this clear, crisp blue sky and white cloudy day, I couldn't help but notice the vast fields of corn and other planted vegetation as we moved on through the next town. There was a vegetable cart with no one attending, but all who stopped by were expected to make a purchase and leave the money. WHAT?! Only in small town USA.

At the town of Choptank the sun beaming down on the huge river and wharf lined with several boats took my breath away. A daring young woman stood on her surfboard at the water's edge and paddled her way about a quarter of a mile to the other side like it was her daily exercise. The town's history on display included the struggles and accomplishments of Frederick Douglass and Harriet Tubman while they were residents and slaves on the Eastern Shore. I went on to Denton to experience the welcoming farm life on over 200 acres of land, with huge tractors, horses, pigs, chickens and rabbits. Thawley's

Chapel, located down the road a piece, offered a nice end (singing "Amazing Grace" and "Oh Happy Day") to an eventful day across the Bay Bridge.

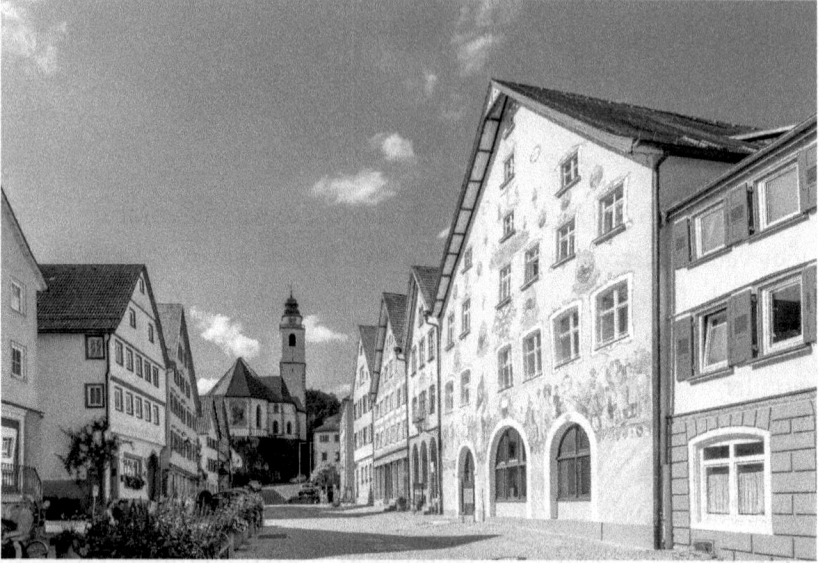

It's Not About You

Some time ago I saw an unusual greeting that said, "I'm sorry. I got angry." Nothing unusual about that, but the picture printed on the card left no doubt to the receiver that their anger left a noticeable dent in the relationship. It displayed a view of an angry man, with an angry face and gnashing teeth, holding a spiked metal club, banging several deep holes into the floor. I am sure the receiver or offended individual, seeing the humor, couldn't resist a laugh or smile. There are many ways to appease anger and lighten the load. However, trying to win back someone who has been offended, particularly among Christian brothers and sisters, takes a little more effort. Before coming to Christ, trying to do and say the right things was a challenge because my heart was not right before God. I learned a valuable lesson some time ago about myself, after feeling offended over a matter. I was ready to throw my hands up and quit the church. Although I felt right in the matter and very sure that the offender needed to change their behavior, I realized there was a need to understand my own emotions and responses and how I was being affected. I was a sister wronged and more unyielding than a fortified city. It turned into an event that was all about ME. Satan, our adversary, was ready to give the "death blow" to my suffering and severely wounded SELF—the coup de grace. I would have, like many, left with unforgiveness in my heart, unwilling to do something to make it right. I realized the need to humble myself and FORGIVE. I don't think God would have heard my prayers over unforgiveness. Although the Bible states be not easily offended, it also makes the point that some are harder to win back than others. "A brother offended is harder to be won than a strong city." I committed to changing my attitude and myself toward the situation, rather than try to force a change in someone else. Once I extended the "olive branch," I was overcome with such peace and love for my friend in Christ. I thank God for a healthy conscience and not giving in to the adversary. I got tested on this recently, being the offender in the matter. And when I realized I caused my friend to be hurt, I immediately asked for forgiveness and let them know that I love them. In either case, do the right thing and make it right with God. We are the peacemakers. Seeking peace and restoration is more important than being right. Disputes are like the barred gates of a citadel. They will have you out in left field, bitter, unyielding and out of God's plan for your life. Protect your prayer life. Embrace forgiveness to experience peace and move forward in what you are called to do in ministry. There is no time to be out of commission. #redeemingthetime

Proverbs 18:19; 1 Corinthians 13: 5, 13; Matthew 5:9; James 3:2

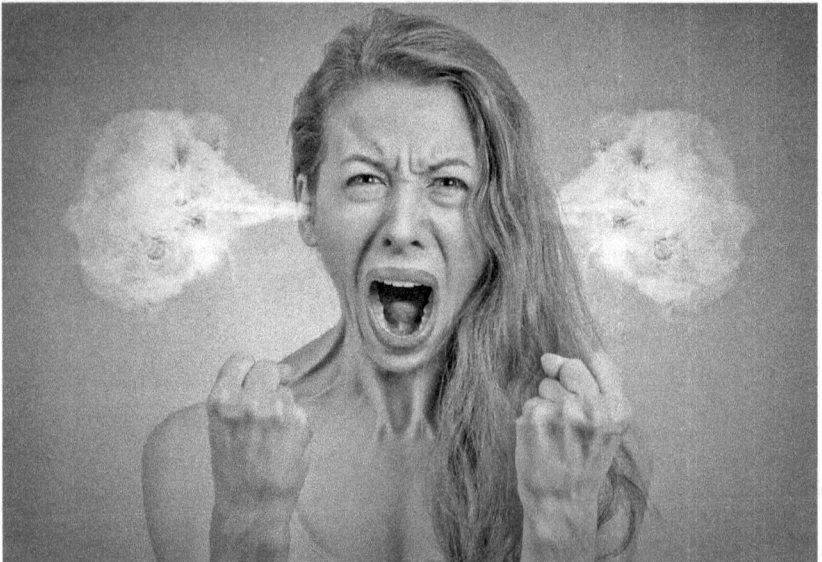

Matter Of Your Soul

Thursday after arriving home from the clinic, I laid down and didn't wake up for the next six hours. Not realizing my phone was on airplane mode, I had missed several calls. I learned later that in that short amount of time our Nation had moved to a National Emergency status.

I believe the Coronavirus has sobered our minds enough to focus on the matter and condition of our soul and spirit. I have had a long time to think about and prepare for the next life. I willingly gave my heart to the Lord way back in 1972. Longevity is a blessing and affords time to make things right with God. If you've never thought about the next life and how to prepare, now is a good time. I love you and want you to reap the benefits of committing your life to the Lord Jesus Christ today. Jesus said " In my Father's House are many mansions: If it were not so, I would have told you. I go to prepare a place for you... that where I am there ye may be also." (John 14:2, KJV)

Repeat this simple prayer. *Lord Jesus, be merciful to me a sinner. Wash me in your blood that you shed for me on the Cross of Calvary. Forgive me of all of my sins. I receive you now as my Savior and I confess you as my Lord.* The Lord hears the prayers of sincere hearts. Begin your journey by reaching out to a place of worship where you will learn to grow as a vessel pleasing to the Lord. You are in my prayers. #redeemingthetime St. John 3:16 - St. John 14:2 - Romans 10:9

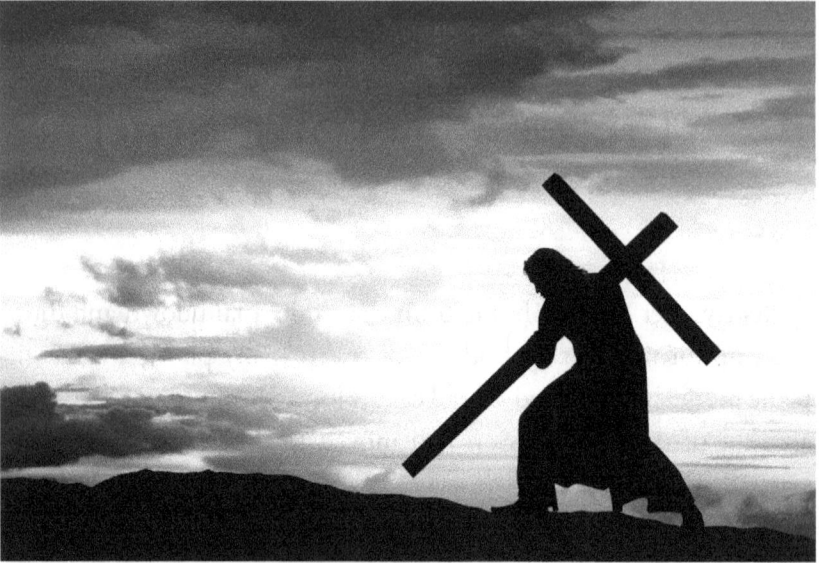

Still In Love?

That alone time, communication, and the constant desire to be in one another's presence reflects how our relationship with the Lord should be. Time spent with the Lord in prayer reflects our confessed love for Him. If He's just an afterthought, or the last on your totem pole of activities, there's something missing in the relationship. Have you found a new love? Have you lost interest? Did you forget how it was when you first fell in love with Him? Renew your commitment to the Lord today. #redeemingthetime.

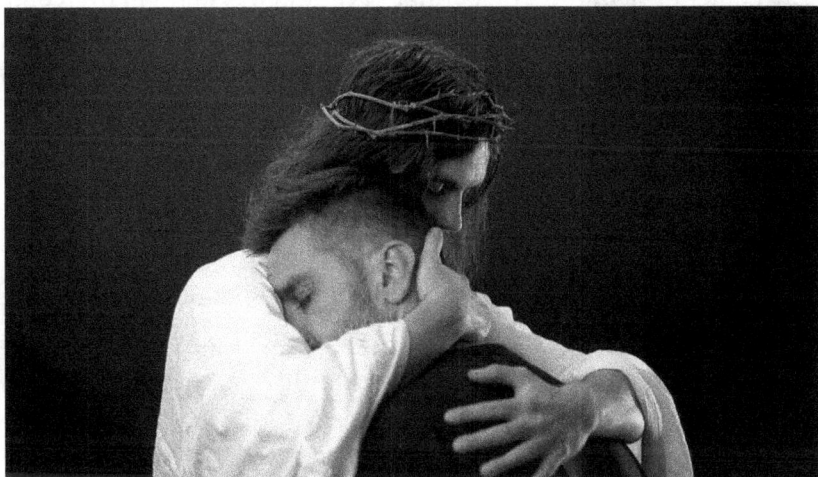

Suffering Persecution

"Yea, and all that will live Godly in Christ Jesus shall suffer persecution." Paul's last letter written from a Roman prison to Timothy reveals his urgent words of counsel. Suffering persecution in those days included torture, whippings, burnings, imprisonment, cruel mocking trials, stoning, being sawn in pieces, being destitute and afflicted, and wandering in deserts, mountains, dens and caves. Paul told Timothy to endure hardness as a good soldier in order to carry on the work of the Lord.

The book of 2 Timothy is sobering. Each time I read it I'm overcome with the feeling of what is most important. What's most important is getting the Word of God, the Gospel of Jesus Christ, and the Good news out to those who don't know. Today we look far off in other countries and see the persecution of Christians, feeling somewhat relieved (due to our legal systems) that it's not happening on our soil. We feel sad for our brothers and sisters and pray continuously for them and their families. Will we be able to stand in that day if it were to happen here? Will we have time to make that phone call and ask for forgiveness? Will we be able to give our lives for our faith in Jesus Christ? #redeemingthetime

Hebrews 11:35-39, 2 Timothy 2:3; 2 Timothy 3:12

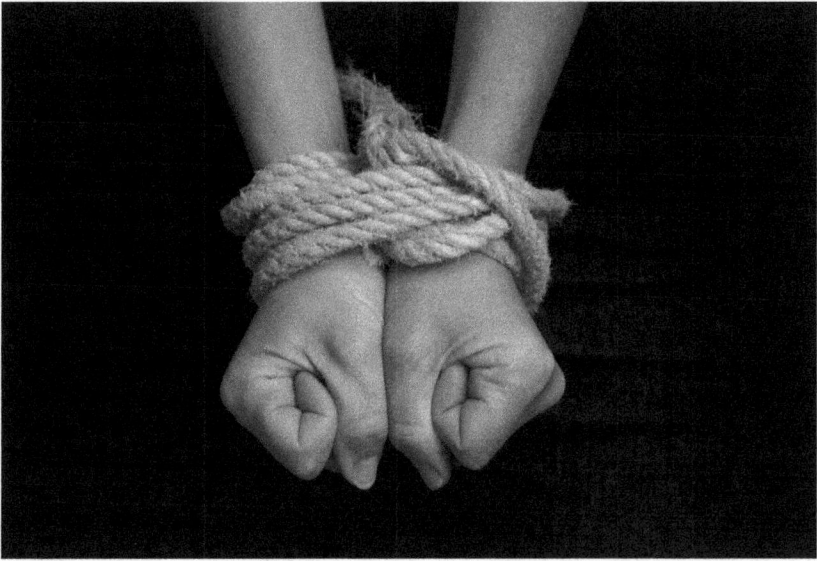

Take Heed

Throughout the ages God has sent many to warn the sinner in their sins. However, God was especially provoked when the sin was among His people in the house of God. In some instances he pointed out to His prophets that the heathen listens and heeds the warnings, but God's people are imprudent, often reproved and stiff-necked.

Ezekiel the prophet was taken up in the spirit by God and was shown what was going on in the house of God that was provoking Him to anger. They were worshipping idols in secret, in dark chambers. In a vision given to the prophet Ezekiel, God had those people marked who were praying against these abominations but poured out His fierce anger on those who said, "God doesn't see, and the Lord has forsaken the earth."

There comes a time when sin has reached the point of God's judgment and He's had enough. In this day and time of worst evils, let's pray that God holds back his judgment, and extends His hand of Mercy to the lost, imprudent, stiff-necked and rebellious. #redeemingthetime

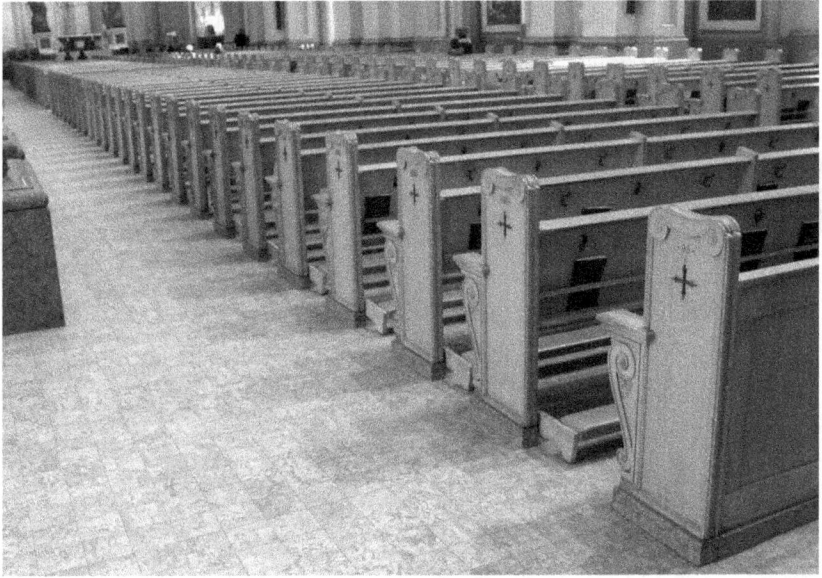

Take The Time

What if? What if we only had a five-minute warning of nuclear missiles headed our way? Or what if a sudden earthquake left no time to run to safety? And, what if the doctor said, "There is nothing more we can do?" In these scenarios, there would be little time to ponder the question, "Where will my soul spend eternity?" The majority of us are busy about life, taking it for granted, overlooking and putting off the need to prepare for the afterlife.

Every person born into this world was meant to live in their natural body forever. Because of one man's sin (Adam), we were all made sinners. And by one man's death on the cross of Calvary (Jesus Christ), we were all given the hope of Eternal Life. Take the time NOW to prepare TO MEET GOD. "For God so loved the world, that He gave his only begotten Son that whosoever believes in Him should not perish but have everlasting life."

IN THE END, Heaven and Earth and all the things in it that take up so much of our attention will pass away. But the Word of God (the Bible) will remain forever. Only the pure in heart will enter into Heaven. GET YOUR HOUSE IN ORDER. Your body is like a tent housing your soul and spirit that is eternal. The way you are living in this life will determine where your soul and spirit will spend eternity. Repent, believe and give your life to Jesus Christ today. #redeemingthetime

Romans 6:12-21; Matthew 24:35; John 3:16; Matthew 5:8; Isaiah 38:1; Romans 10:9; 2 Corinthians 5:1

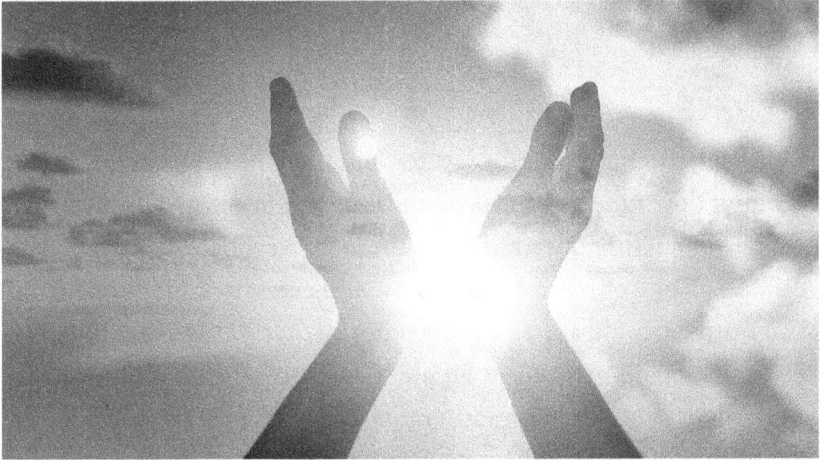

Tears For Mercy

Today has become a hard day for me after hearing the news and scrolling down the various postings on FB. I'm trying to prevent my tears from spilling onto the computer and keyboard as I attempt to respond as one of many voices to the unnecessary killings of African Americans. I could spend all day pointing out statistics that uncover bias and ongoing racism in all areas against my race. However, the resulting debates, opinions and rants alone are enough that fuel and add to the ongoing hate.

Being Black is an honor because of the price that was paid by my relatives and ancestors for my freedom. Research it. We exist and thrive (educated or uneducated) because of the terror experienced just for being Black. Telling a Black person to get over it is like telling the Jew to forget the Holocaust. As in other ethnicities, ethnic cleansings resulting in blood, violence and death mark our histories and are etched in our memories forever. With that said, the hate continues even as I type.

We are Black, here in America, still experiencing terror as the country considers putting up a wall to keep the terror out. Who's going to build the wall for the terror within? It hurts to see and hear that another Black man or woman has been gunned down at the hands of law enforcement or by authorized legal weapons, if you will, as well as dying in custody. The apples-to-oranges comparison is synonymous to the big elephant in the room. When will it end? When Jesus comes and separates the wheat from the tares? In the meantime, what can be put in place to prevent these scenarios? PRAYER IS AT THE FOREFRONT! Reach out to and support those organizations that investigate and hold accountable those responsible for illegal and unnecessary killings of African Americans. #lettherebepeaceonearthandletitbeginwithme

2 Corinthians 10:4-5

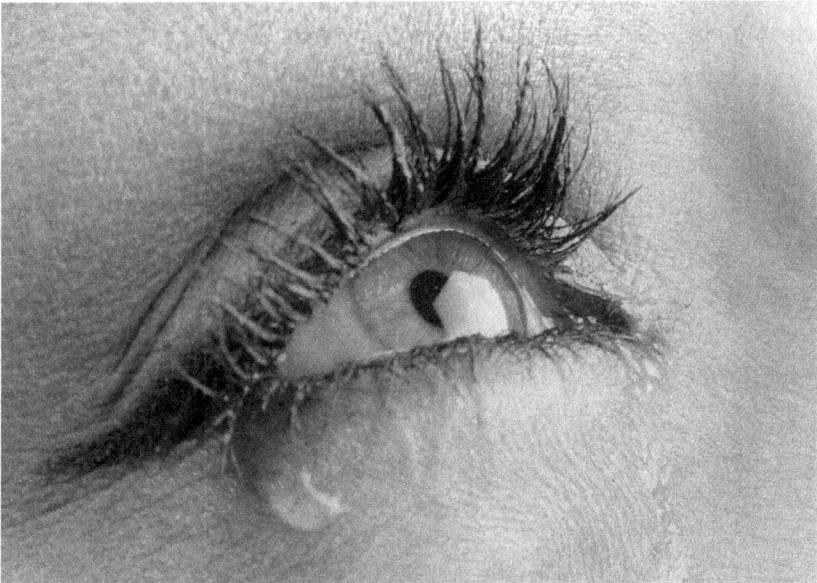

Test Of Love

It was a bitter cold night back in the 90s—much colder than normal. My children were small enough to fit under my coat for protection. We had just left church and were waiting at the bus stop, watching all the familiar faces ride by. I had to catch two buses to get home, where the one dropped us off downtown to wait for the other. Once downtown, I received so many offers from strangers to give us a ride home.

Finally, an off-duty police officer flashed his badge and offered us a ride. However, the bus showed at the same time, after a thirty-minute wait. That's how cold it was that night. Saints of God, let's let our fruit of love and goodness manifest throughout the year. That experience has made me more compassionate for others who find themselves in similar situations.

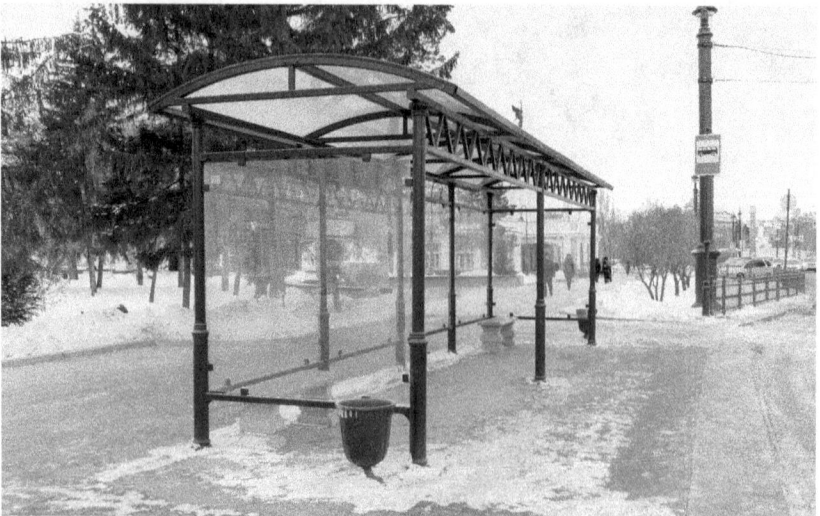

Thankful Prayer

Thank you, Lord, for waking me up to see another day. Some didn't open their eyes today. On this day, dear Lord, make me an example of your love, grace and mercy. Somebody needs you today. Lead me to that one who's crying out in their soul, searching for peace and satisfaction. Let the Good News of your love go forth from these lips one more time.

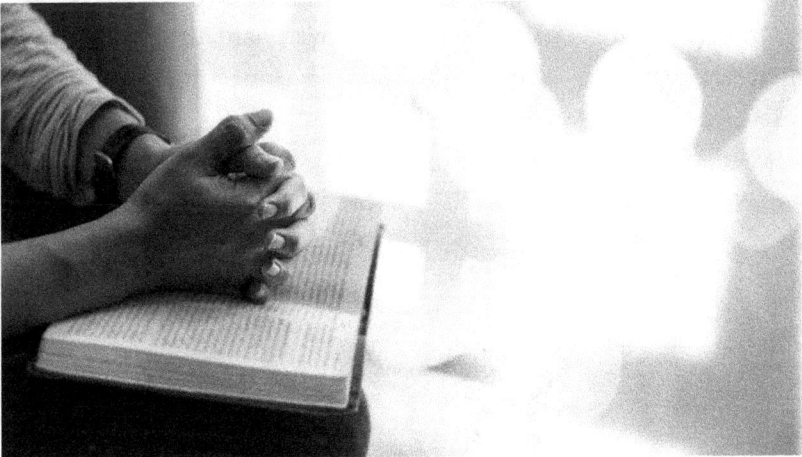

The Battle Is Not Yours

Sometimes our tests and trials can be severe, but God has a purpose. Someone is benefiting from the effects of our storm. The Prophet Jonah was running from God to avoid God's instructions to go preach to a city called Nineveh. He boarded a ship headed in the opposite direction and slept securely as a storm approached. The occupants of the ship became fearful and began calling on their various gods.

When it was discovered that Jonah was running from the presence of the true and living God, he was tossed overboard, and immediately the storm ceased. As a result, the mariners or occupants of the ship feared the God of Jonah, offered sacrifices and made vows to Him. As we learn and continue to allow God to use us, just remember, *the battle is not yours; it's the Lord's.*

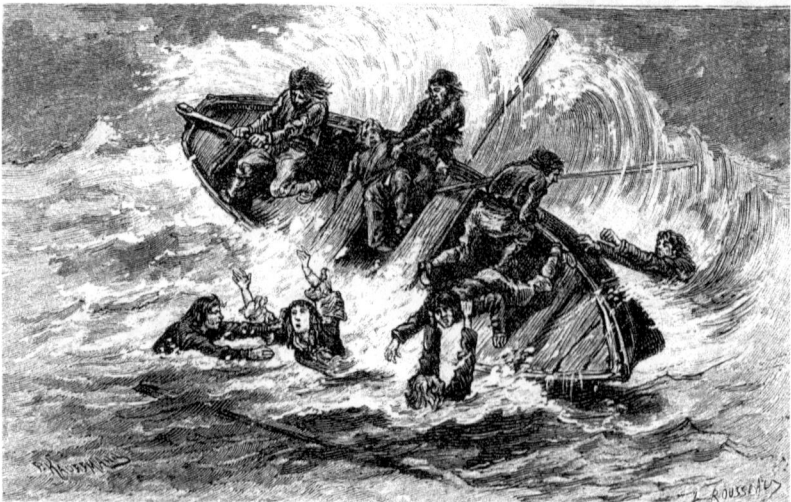

The Bible -
A Great Resource

FOR THOSE WITH QUESTIONS - THE BIBLE IS A GREAT
RESOURCE

"He doth execute the judgment of the fatherless and widow, and
loveth the stranger, in giving him food and raiment." (Deuteronomy
10:18. KJV).

"But the stranger that dwelleth with you shall be unto you as one
born among you, and thou shalt love him as thyself; for ye were
strangers in the land of Egypt: I am the LORD your God." (Leviticus
19:33-34, KJV).

"And if thy brother becomes poor, and falls into decay with thee,
then thou shall relieve him: yea, though he be a stranger, or sojourn-
er; that he may live with thee" (Leviticus 25:35, KJV).

"He that oppresses the poor reproaches his Maker. But he that honors him has mercy on the poor" (Proverbs 14:31, NKJV).

"Wherefore remember, that you being in time past Gentiles in
the flesh, who are called Uncircumcised by that which is called
Circumcision in the flesh made by hands, that at that time you were

without Christ, being aliens from the commonwealth of Israel, and strangers from the covenant of promise, having no hope, and without God in the world" (Ephesians 2:11-12, KJV).

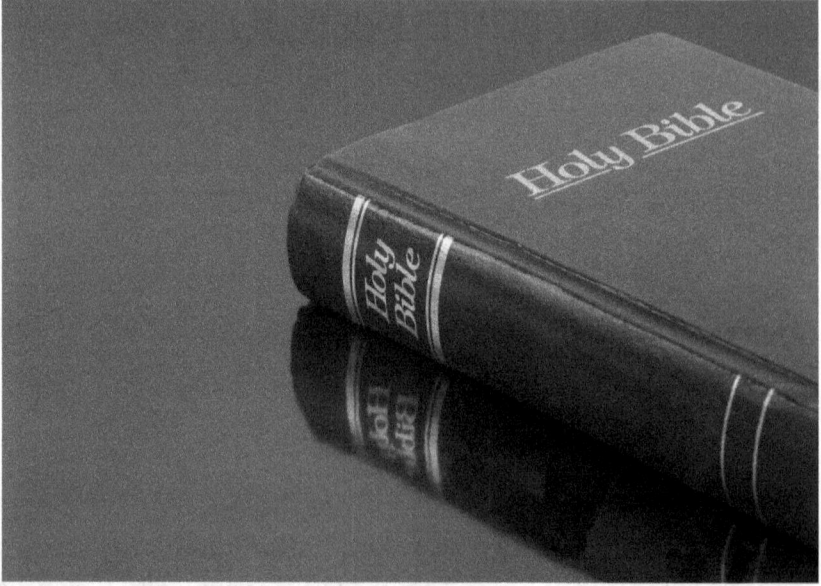

The Commission

Draw me nearer, nearer, blessed Lord... I thought of this song while reading a verse of scripture: "No man can come to me except the Father which has sent me draw him; and I will raise him up at the last day." Jesus made this statement to the Jews who at the time were murmuring about his deity (divine nature). He also stated that every man who has heard and learned of the Father comes to him.

Our witness, teaching, preaching and spreading the Good News are an integral part of the Divine Process for winning souls. The Almighty God and Lord of Hosts is merciful and draws as many as receive His love gift Jesus Christ. #hethatwinssoulsiswise

St. John Chapter 6

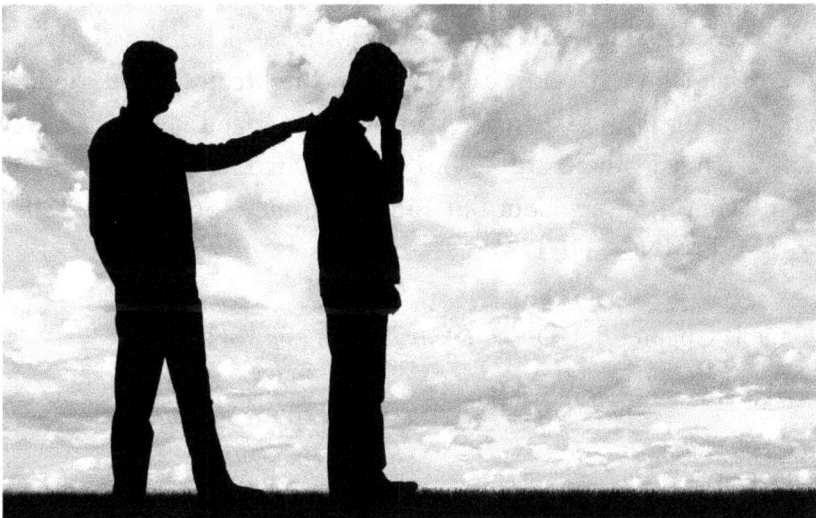

The Father's Business

Abraham challenged God, saying, "Shall not the judge of the earth do right?" because the Lord said, "The cry of Sodom and Gomorrah is great and because their sin is very grievous, I will go down and see whether they have done altogether according to the cry of it, which is come unto me, and if not, I will know." In all of His mercy, God took the time to go down personally. Abraham asked God if he would destroy the righteous with the wicked, even if there were only ten left within the city. God told Him he would not destroy it for the ten's sake. In all His mercy He would have saved the city because of the righteous.

Will God find any righteous when things get as bad as they did in those days? Will He have to come down Himself to observe the situation? Will there be any praying saints left? Will there be anybody on the Lord's side? Will there be any witnesses left telling of God's mercy and love? Because there were no righteous found, Sodom and Gomorrah was destroyed, but not before God's hand of mercy was extended. These are serious times. Our God is still merciful and loving. Let's be about our Father's business. Souls are at stake. #REDEEMINGTHETIME

Genesis Chapter 8; Genesis 19: 1-29; Genesis 18:22-33

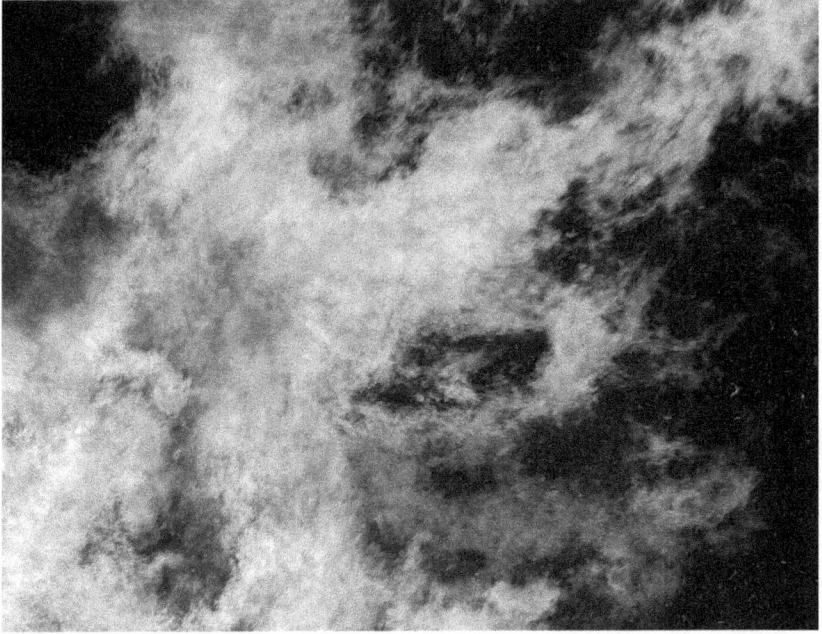

The Heart Of God

I am so GRATEFUL AND HONORED to have been touched by the HEART OF GOD. As one of many experiences, this one stands out in our conversations as significant and timely. It felt like the weight of the world was on me as I prayed and cried. Our God is eager to help us in whatever situation we're in, and is merciful to all. He does not want anyone to perish or be without His love gift to man, JESUS CHRIST OUR SAVIOR.

Even though I was aware of the conversations around me, people leaving in and out of the sanctuary, children playing, etc., it all sounded like a distant roar fading far away. My spirit seemed to soar to some quiet, distant place. Once there, my soul and spirit opened up to God's ear. All I could do was cry and speak unto God. I know He felt my heart and I somehow could sense that He too was grieving for the lost.

There's so much to do in so short a time. The harvest is ripe every-where, right under our noses, in our church outreaches, in our own communities, and on our jobs. REACH OUT AND TOUCH SOMEONE TODAY WITH THE LOVE OF GOD AND THE GOOD NEWS OF SALVATION.

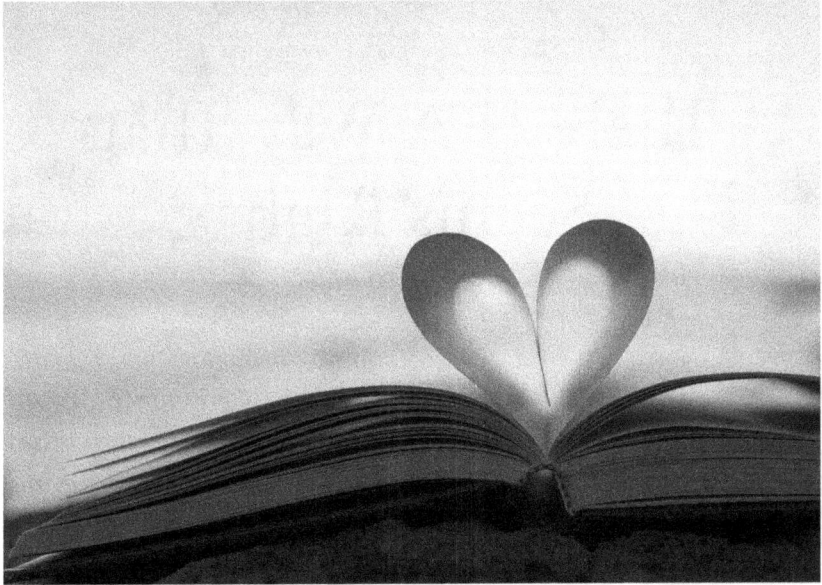

There Is A Way That Seems Right

Pollution is the introduction into the natural environment of contaminants that cause adverse change. We see and experience this in our everyday lives in what we eat and drink and in the air we breathe. So therefore, we take certain precautions to avoid sickness, disease and death. These facts came to mind as I was reading the Biblical account of Sodom and Gomorrah. What moved God to pour out fire and brimstone (sulphur) on whole cities, from the youngest to the oldest? What were the inhabitants doing to bring God to this decision? Where were the preachers and what were the churches doing? How did it get to this point?

The account states that God heard that the sins were very grievous and therefore had to come and see for himself. Abraham asked, "God, would you destroy the cities if there were fifty righteous among them?" God's response was, "If there were even ten righteous, I would not destroy them." Because of the righteousness and prayers of Abraham, his brother Lot and his two daughters were spared. The two destroyers God sent to destroy the cities also came to rescue Lot and his family. They eventually had to blind the homosexuals who were banging at Lot's door trying to have sex with them. Was there some ordinance or unspoken rule in that city stating all male visitors must report to a certain location? Grievous indeed.

Lot had two sons-in-law who refused to leave and a wife who looked back and was turned into a pillar of salt. All the cities were polluted, and I'm sure this didn't happen overnight. In this day and time, we need to be mindful of those things that will attempt to pollute our spirits and souls as we continue to fulfill our commission. We have to take every precaution to guard what's introduced into our spirit. There is a way that seems right to a man, but that way leads to death. We must continue to preach, lift up Jesus and warn the sinners in their sin, even if the whole world says their sin is right. #redeemingthetime

Genesis Chapters 18 &19; Proverbs 14:12

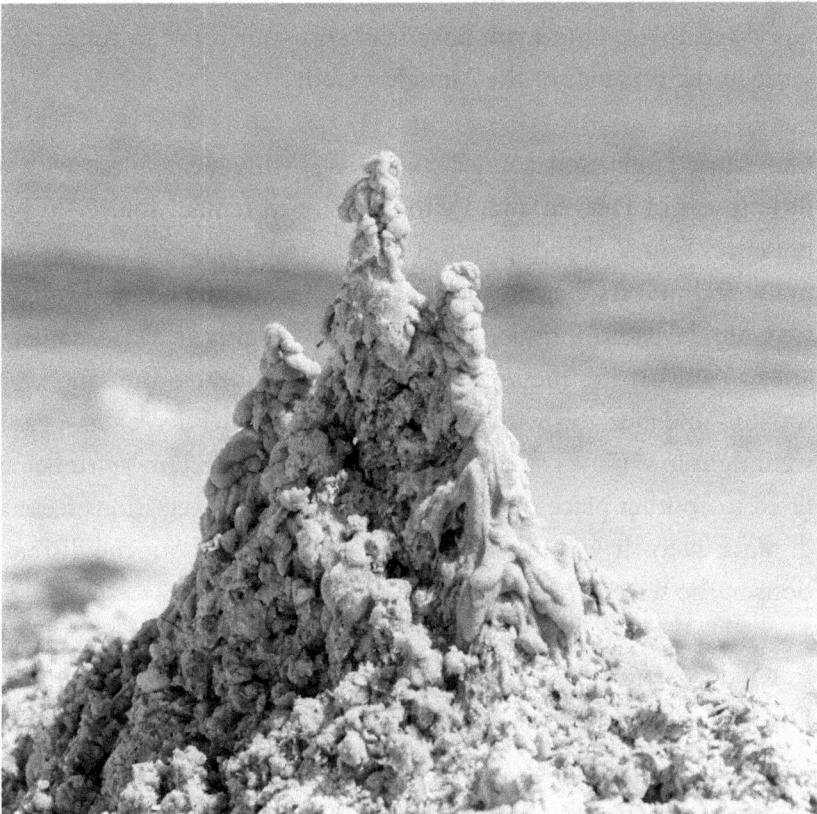

The Secret Place

Our God is a refuge and a fortress. I can go to him and feel peace and safety. There is a place in God for the righteous that the scriptures describe as secret, a place that is engulfed by the shadow of the Almighty God. It is a place where you can be covered completely with the presence of God all around, sweeping over your being like the warmth of a bath towel fresh out of the dryer. Why is this place called secret? It is unknown to others and unseen by others unless you dwell there; unless you have made up your mind to reside and settle in the presence of the Almighty God.

Our Most High God connects with us in this secret place with a little touch of Heaven and a strong desire to remain forever in his presence. Your soul and spirit feel right at home as God receives your praise and prayers, being touched by all that you are going through. One Sunday morning God's presence was mighty in the sanctuary after a soul-stirring message that touched my heart. The sanctuary was full and buzzing with conversation as the service ended. As I went right into prayer where I was seated, I could feel my spirit being lifted to another place that made the buzz and conversations seem a distance away. It was just me and God talking without the distractions in the secret place.

In God's fortress and tower there is safety, security and refuge. Dwelling in the secret place of the Almighty God gets God's attention.

Commit to keeping his attention by dwelling in the secret place every day. #redeemingthetime

Psalm 91:1-4; Proverbs 18:10

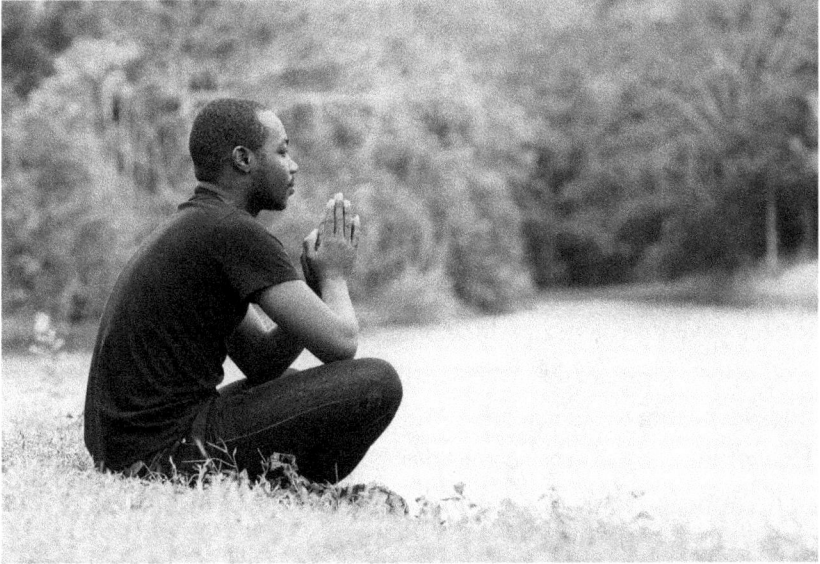

God Wants You

"And I saw a great white throne and Him that sat on it, from whose face the earth and the Heaven fled away. And there was found no place for them. And I saw the dead, small and great, stand before God. And the books were opened, and another book was opened which is the Book of Life. And the dead were judged out of those things that were written in the books according to their works. And the sea gave up the dead which were in it, and Death and Hell delivered up the dead which were in them. And they were judged, every man according to their works. And Death and Hell were cast into the Lake of Fire. This is the second death. And whosoever was not found written in the Book of Life was cast into the Lake of Fire."

John, the servant of Jesus Christ, was exiled to the isle of Patmos and wrote to encourage his fellow Christians as they were facing persecution in Rome. He wrote the visions that were given to him revealing those things that will come to pass.

In our earthly courts, the judge hears testimony and documented facts of the case from representing attorneys. The selected jury listens, a verdict is rendered and the defendant is sentenced or set free as a result. "God so loved the world that he gave His only begotten Son that whosoever believes in Him should not perish but have everlasting life." (John 3:16, KJV) Jesus Christ is our representative here on earth who pleads our case to God the Father and the Judge. The facts are being recorded. What facts? They are your works here on earth. Are you prepared to meet God? Is your name written in the Book of Life? Prepare your soul today. Give Jesus Christ your heart. Confess your sins to Him. Receive Him as your personal Savior and Representative for God. #redeemingthetime

Revelation 20:11-13; John 3:16

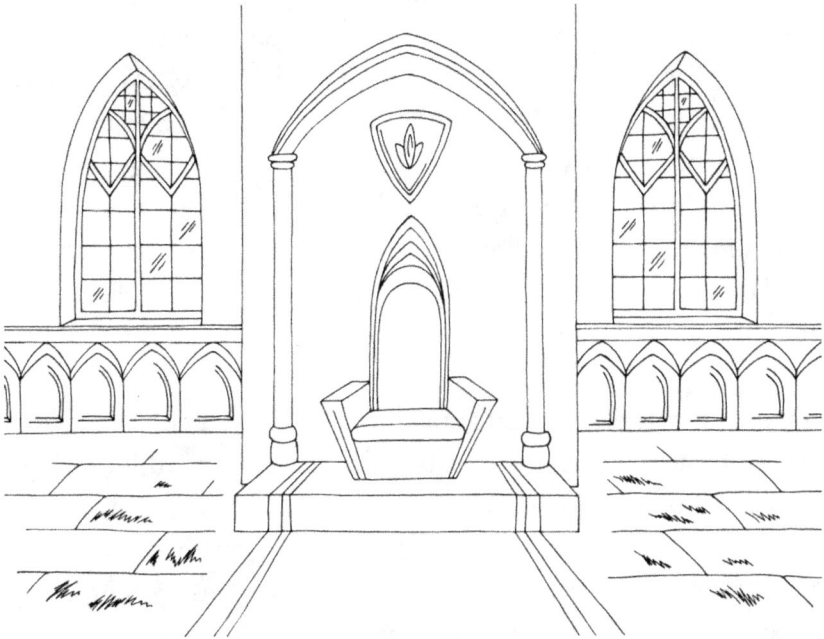

Time Is Short

IT'S TIME! Time to get right with God. It's official, from reputable news media sources that microchips are being implanted under the skin for identification purposes. This is Biblical Prophecy coming to pass that has been preached down through the years, "USHERING IN THE MARK OF THE BEAST 666." IT'S TIME to take heed to what your parents and grandparents have been telling you about getting right with God. IT'S TIME to stop riding on the prayers of others for your soul's wellbeing. You alone will have to stand before God for the deeds you have done on this earth. As a tree falls, so shall it lie. There are no more chances to get it right after death.

Take advantage of God's grace and love TODAY. GIVE HIM YOUR HEART and begin reaping the benefits of a committed life to God. "For God so loved the world that he gave his only begotten Son that whosoever believes in him should not perish but have everlasting life." (John 3:16. KJV) Don't waste time trying to justify your wrong. Be honest. Don't waste time arguing issues and placing blame. Ask Jesus Christ to come into your heart. Ask for forgiveness of all of the sins you've ever committed. He will forgive you.

Whether you understand, believe, or know anything about Biblical Prophecy, realize your very soul is at stake for rejecting Jesus Christ as your Savior. #redeemingthetime

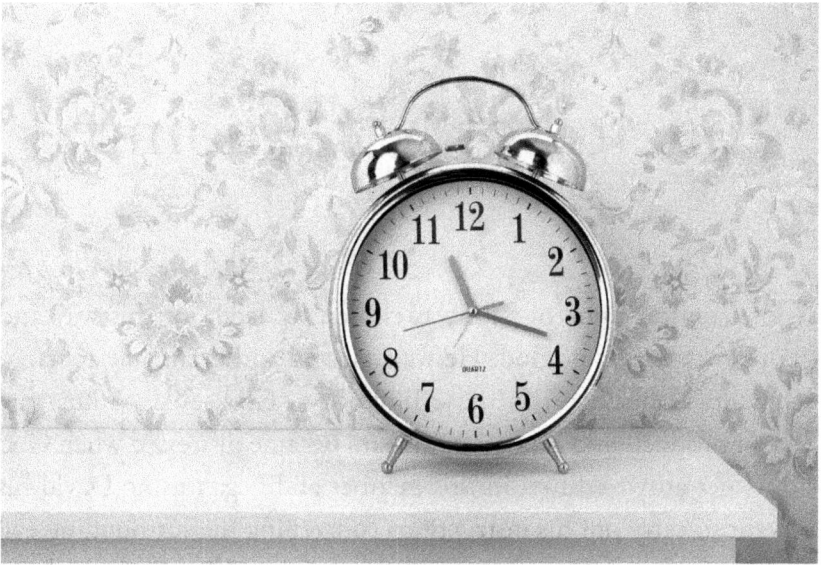

Touch Not My Anointed

A king by the name of Saul was chosen by God, lost his way and became an enemy of God. He was rejected and eventually replaced for being disobedient. In those Bible days, God spoke to kings by way of prophets and dreams. King Saul became distressed when God no longer answered him in this manner and began using David his servant to carry out his instructions concerning the surrounding evil nations. Knowing his replacement was coming, King Saul sought to kill David on several occasions.

The rest of this scenario reveals that God protected David and delivered King Saul into the hands of David. However, when the opportunity presented itself, David chose not to harm the king. He spared his life and bowed before him, later declaring, "Who can stretch his hand against the Lord's anointed and be guiltless?" Because of David's mercy, King Saul acknowledged his wrong and confessed David to be better fit for king. At King Saul's tragic end of life, falling upon his own sword, he requested to be thrust through by a stranger to obtain certain death. When David requested an audience with the stranger and heard his account, David replied, "How were you not afraid to stretch forth your hand to the Lord's anointed? Your mouth has testified against you saying I have slain the Lord's anointed."

David gave respect to King Saul as God's chosen, anointed vessel to the very end of his life. The anointed vessels of God in His church are called unto God's purpose. Let God be their judge. Let's hold them up in prayer. God sees farther up the road and knows the outcome.

#redeemingthetime

Psalm 105:15; 2 Samuel 1:5-16; 1 Samuel Chapter 24; 1 Samuel 26:9; 1 Samuel 26:21; 1 Samuel 28:15

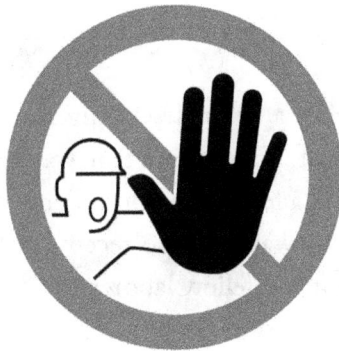

Transformed

On Sunday, February 23rd and in honor of Black History Month, Pastor Sharon Hardy Knotts preached an inspiring, uplifting and heartwarming message of forgiveness and reconciliation.

The Apostle Paul wrote a letter describing himself as a prisoner for Christ and on behalf of Onesimus, a runaway slave accused of theft. Philemon, described as a fellow worker under Paul's ministry and also the owner of the slave, was asked to receive him back with forgiveness, not as a slave but as a fellow laborer in Christ. Paul would have been happy to keep Onesimus with him in light of his conversion and transformation to the Christian faith but considered it better to send him back to effect reconciliation between them as brothers in Christ.

History and ancient tradition reveal that Onesimus went from being a slave to a bishop in Ephesus. This reminds us that biblical characters were real people and were deeply affected by the proclamation of the gospel. They were changed forever and helped others in spite of their circumstances to find freedom in Jesus Christ.

Today, there is still freedom in receiving Jesus Christ into your life. Don't put it off. #redeemingthetime

John 3:16; The book of Philemon; Galatians 3:26

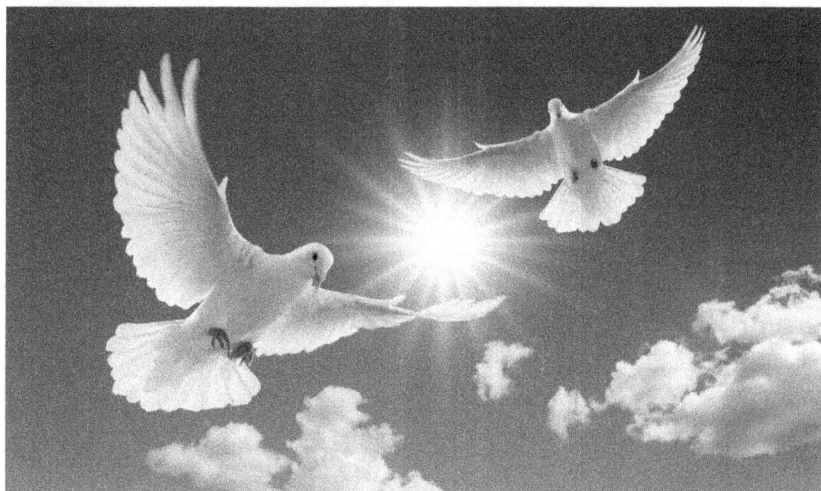

Tribute To Mom

One significant memory about Mom was when she had her church members plan a baby shower for me when I was lonely, pregnant, unmarried and without God. She loved me unconditionally. Mom was kind and always thinking of others. She took care of her surrounding neighbors when she heard they were sick. She never went to bed without kneeling and saying a prayer to God. We didn't have much growing up, but I never heard her complain. She made that fried egg sandwich I took to school for lunch taste so good. The most valuable lesson I learned from her was when she became ill with Alzheimer's Disease, unable to walk or speak. A few days before her death she was smiling and happy. When I fed her one of her final meals, she mouthed the words "thank you." For me that was a gift from Heaven. She is now with the Lord. Mom taught me how to live and how to die. I penned these few words below about her journey in 2010.

As I'm witnessing the transition from death into life, I have to admire the wisdom and love of God in this process. He provides company and conversation, laughter and joyful tears from an unseen world for the dying. As the years of suffering turn into months, weeks, days and into the final hours of this realm, a quiet and serene peace commands the body that seems to ignore its demise. There is no more desire for food or drink or reaching out for assistance. A long and peaceful sleep mixed with slow, silent breaths becomes the daily routine. Something is going on between the soul and its Maker. Intermittently, the arms reach toward Heaven, and return as if disappointed that they didn't reach their destination. God is steadying my hand as I proceed to provide the day's ADLs in the midst of His work in progress. The hair, the nails, and all that surround must be presentable for an audience with the King. That's what Mom would have wanted.

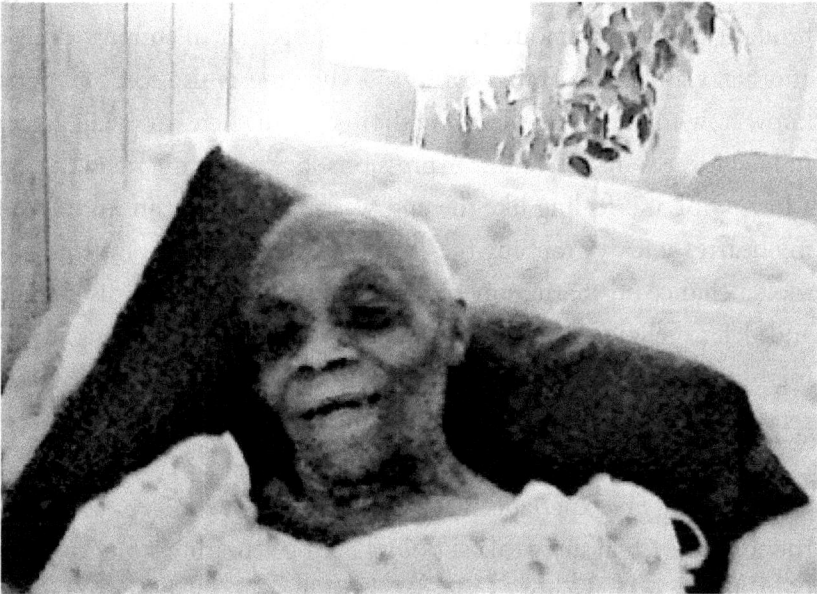

Trust God

A friend asked, "How do I go out gracefully?" Terminal illnesses have brought patients from around the globe together in support of one another via various online forums. "My time is limited." "I don't know how to die." "Are there any thoughts out there on dying gracefully?" These were a few more expressions spoken by my friend during a low point and feeling like the end was near that put an urgency in my heart. Quickly grabbing the opportunity, and with compassion, I took a chance on sharing my faith. These types of forums discourage and delete religious conversations, scripture quoting and encouraging others to adhere to a particular faith. Nevertheless, a soul was at stake and needed an intervention.

First, sharing my experience with the same health concern, I told my friend that even at my weakest points I am celebrating strength from God, and that I have hope in Jesus Christ his son, the Hope of Glory. "I gave my life to Jesus Christ the son of God many years ago, to live in obedience to him for the rest of my life. Knowing that God has prepared a place for those who love him and should he call me home, I am at peace. I will transition from death to eternal life to live forever." I prayed over these words, that they would not be deleted, and that God would touch my friend's heart and complete what could not be shared. TO GOD BE THE GLORY. THE COMMENTS WERE NOT DELETED!

Two negative responses followed. I was told not to give any credit to the supernatural, but rather to hard work, tenacity and good medical practice. And I was told to keep my religious dogma private, that it was cruel and absurd! SAINTS OF GOD, AIN'T NOBODY MAD BUT THE DEVIL! Please keep my friends in prayer.

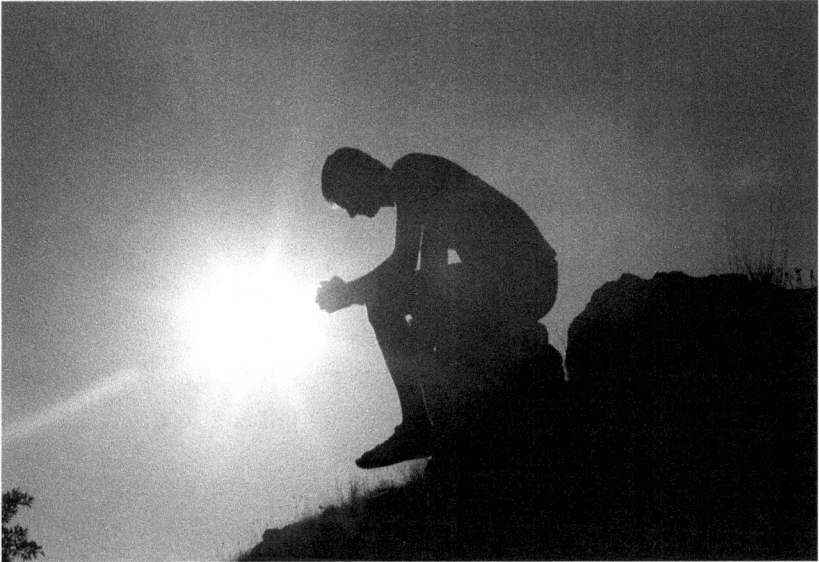

Trust God's Plans

Not taking counsel or seeking direction from the Lord on major concerns can affect many people; particularly if the Lord has given you previous direction about the matter. Joshua was faced with a situation that needed the Lord's attention, but the matter was settled with an oath in the Lord's name instead. The outcome ended in tragedy "down the road" with the killing of seven people not directly involved. Now there were Kings united in purpose to fight against Joshua and Israel. Joshua was instructed by God to lead his armies to overtake these Kings and their cities with His help. This news spread across many lands causing fear, prompting the inhabitants of Gibeon to devise a clever plan. For their protection and safety, they came up with a bogus Peace Treaty (to be in league with). Joshua agreed with the Treaty and made peace with the Gibeonites. The Princes of the Congregation as well promised the safety of the Gibeonites without consulting the Lord. It was later discovered by Joshua that they were indeed neighbors of the Israelites and not from a far country as mentioned. As a result, Joshua cursed them turning them into hewers of wood, bondsmen and drawers of water. However, they were still safe from destruction. In those days a man's word was better than a contract which bound the entire Congregation against harming the Gibeonites.

Now here comes Saul, who is zealous for the children of Israel and murders a remnant of the Gibeonites during King David's reign. This angered God causing a judgement of famine in the land for three years. King David in an attempt to restore the relationship with the Gibeonites grants retribution and delivered to them seven of Saul's sons for execution (hanging).

Out of this study comes several lessons. Lesson #1: Seek the Lords' direction in all aspects of my life. If counsel and direction was sought from God, seven people would not have died in the latter scenario. Lesson #2: Respect who the Lord has put in charge. God knows how to deal with those he has chosen if they step out of line. Lesson #3: Respect what God has allowed. Saul overlooked David's leadership and the fact that God was okay with the safe relationship between the Gibeonites and the Israelites. God called Saul's murder rampage, a "bloody house", causing many people to be in a famine for three years.

A zeal without knowledge can wreak havoc in many lives in and out of the church. It seems a lot of things went wrong from the very beginning. Failing to seek counsel from God can create a "snowball effect." Trust God's plans. #redeemingthetime #oldtestamentadmonitions

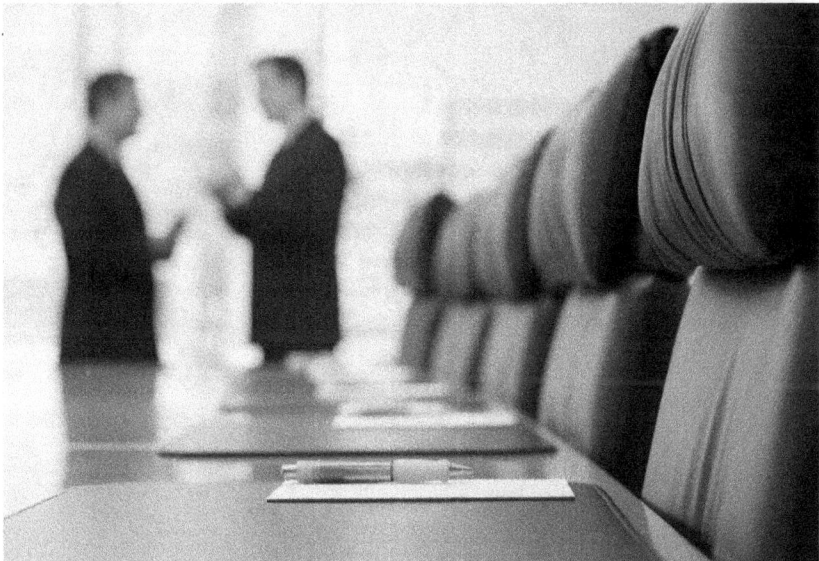

Trust The Outcome

Trusting God means knowing that God's plans are the best plans and He knows what's around the corner and up the road. There are many reasons why things happen in our lives, but we have a God who can turn our dark days and deepest valleys into glorious outcomes. Sometimes we cry and ask "why?" God knows all about your situation and, according to his plans, the outcome will bring glory to Him and knowledge to others that He exists and is real. #redeemingthetime

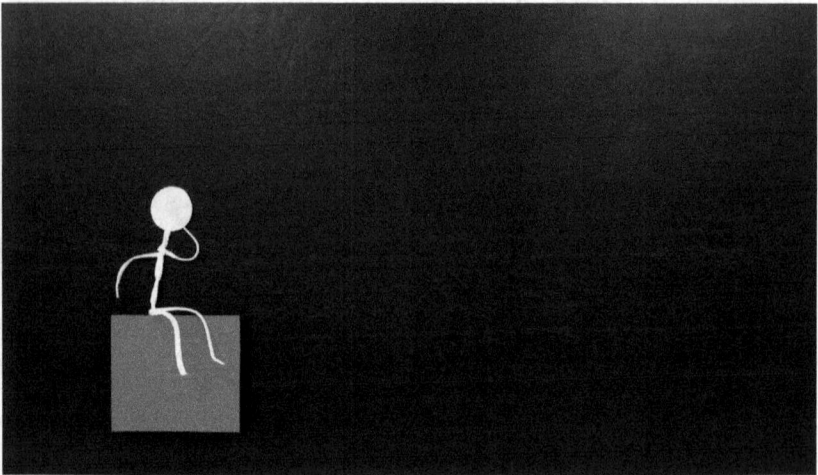

Turn On The Spotlight

"If I regard iniquity in my heart, the Lord will not hear me" is a statement David made while expressing his love for God. He realized through experience that there were just some things he could not do if he was to remain connected to God. He knew God would not listen to his prayer or his praise if he held on to sin in his heart.

God searches all hearts and understands all the imaginations of the thoughts. David encouraged his son Solomon to seek and serve God with a pure and perfect heart. God chose Solomon, a young and inexperienced man, to build a house for the sanctuary. He was also encouraged to go forward with God's plan and to be strong.

Our God chooses and plans his purpose in us. He expects us to carry out his plan out of a pure heart. We encounter many bridges and bumps along the way, but our God is merciful. David said, "God heard me. He attended to the voice of my prayer. Blessed be God which has not turned away my prayer, nor his mercy from me." #redeemingthetime

Psalm 66:18 - 20; 1 Chronicles 28:9,10;1 Chronicles 29:1

Unity In Troubled Times

Thank you, Father, for hearing and answering our collective prayers to spare lives in the wake of potentially devastating hurricanes, floods, fires, tornadoes and earthquakes. Thank you for the change in direction by your mighty hands, the weakening in strength of nature's powerful forces and saving lives. Thank you for touching hearts and providing financing for relief efforts in all affected areas as well as the island territories.

In these few weeks we have become a family that prays together, works together, cries together, hopes together, gives together and loves together. But most importantly, we have become a family that acknowledges your sovereignty as the One who hears and answers prayer. In these few weeks, a mountain of issues was put on hold as we came together to help each other. Thank you, Heavenly Father, for your faithfulness, in the name of Jesus.

ON THIS 9/11 ANNIVERSARY, and as lives slowly return to normalcy, don't forget the kindness and mercy of God. Let us all commit to turning our lives around to stay focused on those things that are important.

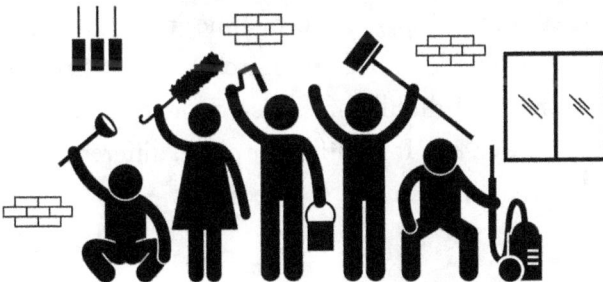

Walk Circumspectly

The callings, the offices, the positions and the titles that the Lord entrusts to us should not be handled lightly. When God qualifies us to be used of Him, he expects us to follow Him in obedience to His Word and as examples of righteousness.

Eli was a priest of God, chosen in succession to his father the priest. He was commanded by God that his household should offer up yearly sacrifices for the people of God upon the altar of God in the taber-nacle, and to walk before Him forever. As the years passed by, and Eli grew old, the people of the congregation became disgusted with going up yearly to offer their sacrifices. The sons of Eli who served under him were threatening and forcing the people to give them the best part of their sacrifices to be used to satisfy their own lust. They were also causing many of them to sin before God by lying with the women at the tabernacle door. This practice went on until God said it was enough. A man of God came to Eli with a rebuke from God, saying, "You have honored your sons above God by allowing them to continue to do evil in the tabernacle."

As in this realm and dispensation of time, these same practices are happening all over the world in churches everywhere. The media keeps us aware of all the ills of Christendom: scandals, pedophilia, greed, pride, power, etc. It's a different place, different people, differ-ent titles, but the same sin and disobedience.

In my recent studies, I've learned that God allows space for repentance. Eli was old and well into his calling when God rebuked him. The sons were unrepentant and refused to listen to their father. Eli should have removed them from their positions in the tabernacle at some point. In another example, Saul pursued the Gibeonites three years outside of the will of God, killing them, although they were approved by God to live peaceably among the Israelites. The judgments of God in these cases were severe. Eli was reduced in strength. God told him, "All the increase of thine house shall die in the flower of their age."

David inquired of God about the three-year famine in the land. God told him it was because of Saul's murderous rampage against the Gibeonites. David could have used his position to stop Saul. Saul's sons were also hanged due to his actions. It pays to obey God, particularly those in positions of authority and leadership over God's people. We cannot and should not frustrate the grace of God, knowing that He sent his love gift Jesus Christ to redeem us back to Him. Now we can thank God that because of Christ, if we do sin, He is faithful and just to forgive us. God knows our hearts and knows what we will do before we do it. The scenarios in the Old Testament are for our admonition and warning and help us to walk circumspectly.

I thank God for the foundation of the Word of God from a place that instructs and teaches the whole counsel of God. More importantly, I thank God for being among people who walk and live according to the Word before the people of God.

1 Samuel Chapter 2; 2 Samuel Chapter 22

What's Happening Lord?

I was standing at the window of my high school classroom watching the sky turn into a red, orange and yellow sunset. We were working on the school yearbook, spending a few hours after school for the same. It was a troubling week for me because the Cuban Missile Crisis was dominating the news media, catching the entire world's attention as well as my own. Imagining a missile exploding creating a fiery image 10 times that of a sunset gave me a sick feeling in my stomach. Fear and dread plagued my mind each day during that national crisis. I wanted to turn the TV off and at the same time keep it on, wanting to know what was going to happen next. My ears were not tuned into the political ramifications during that time to piece together some understanding of the matter. All I could think of was the imminent threat of war, destruction and death. I did not want to die.

So here we are again, in a serious and fragile national crisis. In January, we were on the edge of war. One week, one day and one word could have changed our lives forever. Less than two months later we find ourselves in a worldwide pandemic. Added to this current crisis is also worldwide civil unrest. God is watching and is in control. I believe the Book of Remembrance is opened and recording our responses to these events. What if we found ourselves faced with imminent danger? Would we abandon our political debates, talking points and arguments, or would we take inventory and try to get our houses in order? Would an event such as these drive us to consider where our souls will spend eternity? Would we make things right with God or show concern over where others will spend eternity? Would we have time to ask forgiveness of someone we offended? At the age of 17, I didn't know God enough to consider these questions during the Cuban Missile Crisis. I was too busy worrying about dying.

Today, I can completely trust God with my life, without fear or dread of anything. I asked God to forgive me of all of my sins and committed my whole life to his will. God is in control of everything and will always hear your prayer upon meeting his will for your life. Give yourself to Jesus Christ your Savior. Repent and commit yourself to his will. Trust him with your life. He will give you peace in the midst of any crisis. "For God so loved the world that he gave his only begotten Son, that whosoever believes in him should not perish but have everlasting life." #redeemingthetime

John 3:16

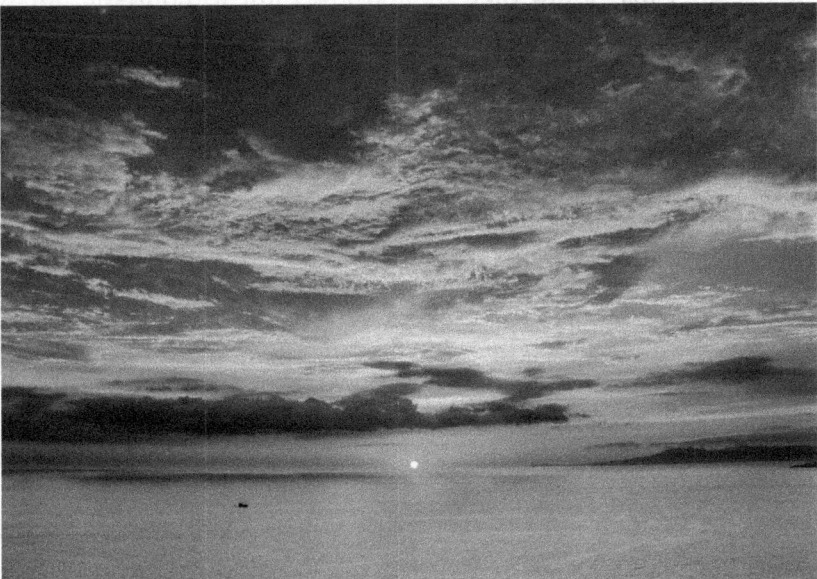

World Crisis Prayer

I don't know which tragedy to pray for first. It's everywhere: at home, here in America, and abroad. I'm having tears for breakfast this morning. Sometimes the Lord lets you feel what's going on inside those who are suffering. So many lives lost (over 10,000) in Nepal. The survivors need our prayers.

Christians are being killed in multitudes in the Middle East. The survivors need our prayers. People and homes are being swept away by floodwaters and tornadoes. Murders are on the increase and happening worldwide. The survivors need our prayers, saints. Oh Lord, when they question You and ask why, reveal Yourself to them mightily that they may know they are hopelessly lost without You. Draw them nigh and closer to You when the heart is tender and sincere. Send Your Word and draw them to a place of understanding concerning Your purpose, in Jesus' name.

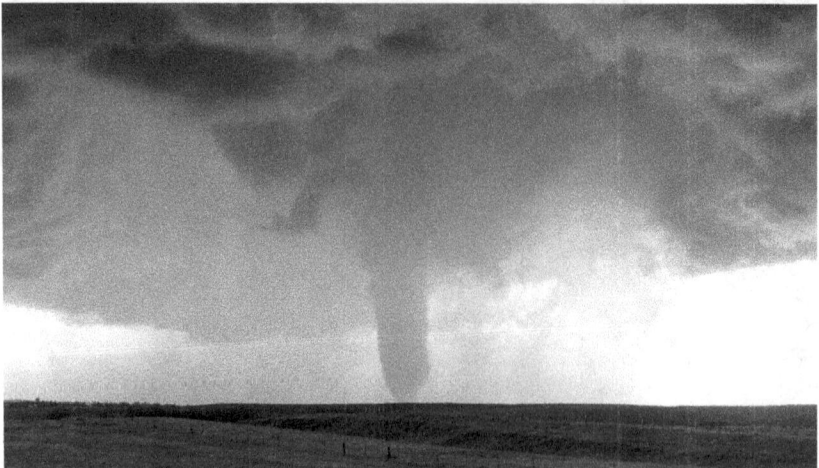

Your Will Be Done

I'm thanking my Heavenly Father for a new year of life in 2017. I'm asking him to increase my love for all mankind, to let me see them as he sees them. It's easy to love the lovable. The test and task comes when reaching out to, interacting with and extending the olive branch to those who oppose themselves, and are dealing with many issues. In some cases, professional help is needed. But first I have to turn the spotlight on myself, to be careful not to judge those who do not receive the words of Christ. The Apostle Paul had the huge task of caring for the people of the many churches that were established by him, as well as the responsibility of representing Christ and being the example as he preached to others.

He wrote many letters to encourage them as they were growing in Christ and was careful not to offend the unregenerated, who opposed Christ. I have to look beyond the fault and see the need of those whose souls are crying out but don't realize the need for the Savior. I am endeavoring to always be in the right place spiritually for the Lord to show me and let me feel these needs.

Let the words of my mouth and the meditations of my heart Lord be acceptable in your sight. #redeemingthetime

Psalm 19:14; John 12:47; Acts 24:16; Acts 25:1-12; 1 Corinthians 15:58

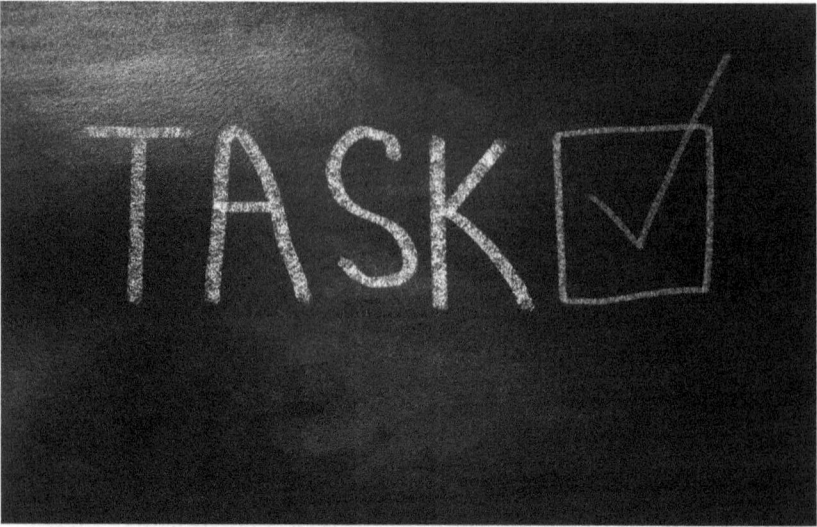

Made Perfect In Weakness

I spent some time in the tuning and R & R station, better known as the hospital, yesterday and today. It was the second time in the past two months being treated for unrelated cancer issues that have not been a problem for many years. Most of you know my story as a survivor of Multiple Myeloma Bone Cancer for the past six years. In the midst of this health journey God has been gloriously moving by his spirit in my life. I am feeling his closeness more than ever before.

On each of these two visits, I met a Christian who shared words of encouragement and prayers, and at the same time was able to share the love of Christ. The trials of our faith, no matter how severe, can bring hope and inspiration to others reaching out for answers about their own health crisis.

As we trust and believe God for positive outcomes and stand on his Word, our faith is being exercised. Our adversary is not happy that despite his subtle attacks on God's people, souls are being inspired and encouraged in the Lord. I refuse to lie wounded on the battle-field indefinitely and complain that the war is unfair. I will continue to rise up in the name of the Lord, move forward and fight the good fight of faith.

Sometimes we stop and ask why and fall into discouragement. But God always has someone in the midst of the battle to bring an encouraging word. Trust God to continue strengthening you in your weakness. His strength is made perfect in your weakness.

"And he said unto me, My grace is sufficient for thee: for my strength is made perfect in weakness. Most gladly therefore will I rather glory in my infirmities, that the power of Christ may rest upon me." (2 Corinthians 12:9, KJV). #redeemingthetime

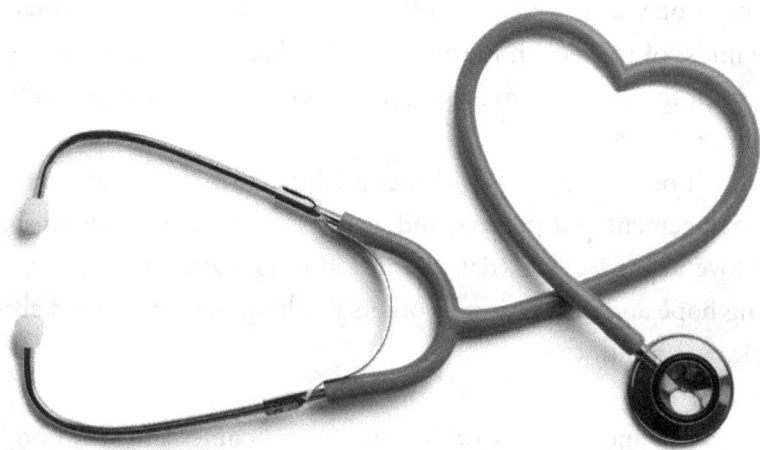

Quotes After Diagnosis (Multiple Myeloma) 2011

Met with the neurosurgeon today. The area of concern on the spine is stable. No surgery! GOD IS ABLE! Come on and praise Him with me, saints!

A smile accomplishes much more than a stare. Give someone a smile today.

At work counting my blessings and sharing the gospel one more time.

Thanking God for new strength today.

Up managing pain. Thank you for your help, Lord.

Our tests only come to make us strong. Trust God at His Word today. (1 Peter 1:6-7).

Walking in the shoes of the severely tested? Stand. Be steadfast, unmovable, always abounding in the work of the Lord.

About the Author

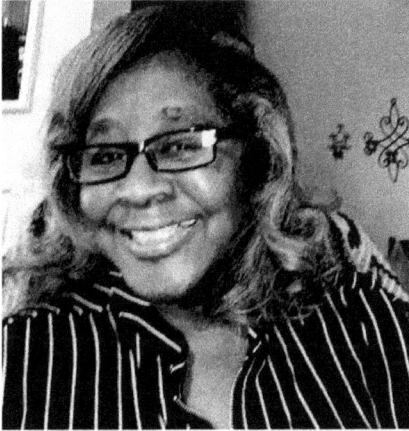

Noble Brun

Turning lemons into lemonade was not a quick decision at the onset of my Multiple Myeloma diagnosis. Mom had passed away after seven years of in-home care, and a deserving labor of love it was. That following year I began to experience pain off and on in and around my rib cage. The pains grew stronger and longer, eventually landing me in the ER seeking treatment. That night the wait for an answer was longer than usual, judging from previous visits. Finally, two physicians met with me to go over the results of the tests that were previously ordered. One physician held the microfilm against the lighted panel while the other physician pointed out the diagnosed problem. She advised as she pointed out certain areas that I had some type of cancer going on and to follow up with an oncologist. There was a moment of silence and a quickening of peace that washed over me before I could respond or speak.

"I had a little talk with Jesus and told him all about my troubles.

"Is that all?" my youngest son replied when I gathered my children to reveal the report and prognosis from the doctors. Five years was the standard life expectancy at that time for patients with Multiple Myeloma bone cancer.

I've learned over time that when God brings you to a situation, good or bad, you won't be walking alone. It has been nine years and counting with trusting God and leaving the outcome in his hands. That has been working for me enough to concern myself with living, loving, and sharing the love of God. He is a help in the time of need.

Many thanks to the staff and physicians at Johns Hopkins Hospital Sidney Kimmel Cancer Center for all they are doing in the treatment of Multiple Myeloma bone cancer and other blood cancers.

To God be the glory for the Great Physician Jesus Christ, who took our infirmities and bore our sicknesses via 39 stripes for all manner of disease at the Cross on Calvary. In Him do I put my ultimate trust.